ENERGY DRAINERS
ENERGY GAINERS

Other books by Paul C. Reisser

Help for the Post-abortion Woman
(with Teri Reisser)

SOLUTIONS TO CHRONIC FATIGUE

ENERGY DRAINERS

ENERGY GAINERS

PAUL REISSER, M.D.

PYRANEE BOOKS

Zondervan Publishing House
Grand Rapids, Michigan

Energy Drainers, Energy Gainers
Copyright © 1990 by Paul Reisser

Pyranee Books
Published by Zondervan Publishing House
1415 Lake Drive, S.E., Grand Rapids, Michigan 49506

Library of Congress Cataloging-in-Publication Data

Reisser, Paul C.
   Energy drainers, energy gainers / Paul Reisser.
    p. cm.
   ISBN 0-310-53971-4
   1. Fatigue. 2. Chronic fatigue syndrome. I. Title.
RB150.F37R45 1990
616.85′28—dc20   90–12691
                                               CIP

Edited by Linda Vanderzalm
Designed by Kim Koning

Printed in the United States of America

90 91 92 93 94 95 / LP / 10 9 8 7 6 5 4 3 2 1

*To the many people in my practice
who are coping with chronic fatigue
and from whom I've learned so much*

Contents

-*Acknowledgments*-

Like nearly every part-time author, I wrote this book during the "cracks" in the day (or more often, the night) after work hours, family time, and other everyday duties were completed. During the final weeks of preparation, however, those cracks became more cavernous, and I need to publicly thank my wife, Teri, and my children, Chad and Carrie, who put off more than a few activities until the final manuscript was in the mail.

Paul C. Reisser, M.D.
February 1990

PART I
WHY AM I SO TIRED ALL THE TIME?

ONE
The (Usually) Unanswered Question

The phones have been jammed with calls from people aching from this year's edition of the flu. The waiting room is full, and the patients just arriving are hearing that the office is running forty-five minutes behind schedule. Mr. Nelson has just had his blood pressure checked and an incidental wart frozen. This didn't take very long, and his doctor is mentally calculating the unexpected catch-up time now available. As the conversation draws to a close, Mr. Nelson nervously clears his throat and utters the most dreaded phrase in medicine: *"By the way . . ."*

Those three words signal the actual agenda for the visit. The suspense is building. What does Mr. Nelson really want to talk about? An unusual pain somewhere? A rash? Headaches? Actually a question about a specific disease wouldn't be too bad. A fever, chest pain, or a worrisome lump will pique the doctor's curiosity or even generate a little rush of adrenaline if something *really* interesting is going on. This is especially true if the problem is clearly visible, and even more so if something can be done about it.[1]

Why Am I So Tired All the Time?

Instead, Mr. Nelson's question is not about a specific disease but about life, from one end of the day to the other: "Why am I so tired all the time?" Unfortunately, his question can't be answered in a few minutes, if it can be answered at all.

George, eighty-five, has recently recovered from a shattering hip fracture that has reduced his stride to a shuffle behind a walker.[2]

He lives with his son's family, fortunate indeed to be kept in the mainstream of family relationships rather than in the kind but dreary ghetto of a nursing home. His grievances ricochet off one another:

"I feel so lousy all the time."

"Why do I get so dizzy?"

"I wake up halfway through the night and can't go back to sleep."

"Could you give me something to pep me up?"

Brenda, thirty-four, is the mother of a twelve-year-old from a previous marriage and three children under age five from her current one. Her husband gives her no particular cause for grief, the bills are paid more or less on time, and no one in the family is ill. But Brenda can hardly get out of bed in the morning.

"I'm more tired when I get up than when I go to bed."

"I've cut way back on sugar, but it hasn't helped."

"Do you think I need vitamins?"

The (Usually) Unanswered Question

Chuck, thirty-eight, has been gradually feeling more fatigued for the past few months. He sprays paint on cars all day at a local body shop, usually consuming a six-pack in the process. Getting his work done isn't much of a problem, but if he climbs a flight of steps or tries to mow the lawn, he feels as if his battery just went dead. If he rests for a little while, he feels okay—until he tries to do the same thing again.

"I can pay a neighborhood kid to mow my lawn, but he can't climb stairs for me."

"I know I need exercise, but that's when I feel the worst."

"Do you think I should cut back on the beer?"

Claudia is raising her two sons single-handedly, negotiating real estate deals, and participating in school and church activities as well. Her day begins at five o'clock in the morning and ends seventeen hours later, during which she tries to overcome both her tiredness and a headache that looms like a thundercloud.

"I feel exhausted and overwhelmed, like I'm going to sink."

"After I fall asleep for a couple of hours, I keep waking up all night long."

"One of my friends has Epstein-Barr virus infection, and her symptoms were just like mine."

Carolyn has no children and is on the verge of having no marriage as well. Her husband has moved out, and her family lives far away. She is learning stenography, but otherwise she has few outside activities and little energy.

"I take plenty of vitamins, but I still feel drained."

"I can't seem to lose any weight, and I don't like the way I look."

"My counselor thought I'd better be checked to make sure I don't have a medical problem."

Every day physicians see thousands of people with chronic tiredness as their primary concern, even though something else is the stated complaint.[3] Millions more plod along, as they have for weeks or months, hoping that tomorrow will bring more energy. Some seek answers from the fringes and frontiers of health care, looking to exotic diets or unusual therapies to provide some improvement. Rich or poor, busy or bored, young or old, the person who comes to the doctor because of tiredness will probably experience something like the following scenario.[4]

The physician will ask questions about specific symptoms, perform a physical examination, and order blood, urine, and other studies if appropriate. When all is said and done, poked and prodded, reviewed and evaluated, the exhausted person will almost always hear this long-awaited verdict: "I don't find much wrong with you."

For some people, this is good news. *Whew! No anemia, diabetes, hepatitis, kidney failure, cancer, or AIDS. My nightmares about suffering, disability, and financial ruin can stop. Thank you, Lord. Thank you, doctor. Now I can get on with life!*

The (Usually) Unanswered Question

For others, the reaction is just the opposite. *All this money and time spent and still no answer. What do I do now? Should I ask for more tests? Should I get a second opinion? If only the doctor would give me a pill to end this fatigue.*

A small number of tired patients will hear a different response: "I've gone over all your results, and as best I can see it looks as if you have . . ."

I need further tests? What kind of a scan? You want me to see Dr. who? Is he some kind of surgeon, or what? Am I going to need to do all this in the hospital?

For a few, the diagnosis of a genuine medical problem gives them great relief. *Well, at least it wasn't all in my head.*

Most tired people who seek answers in their doctors' offices will not leave with a specific, treatable diagnosis—an outcome that some will find reassuring and others exasperating. Whether or not ideas are offered to help resolve the fatigue will depend on the expectations of the patient and the inclinations of the doctor. All too often, there is barely enough time to offer more than reassurance: "Whatever it is, it isn't fatal." From a practical standpoint, even the most caring physician will be hard-pressed to look very far beyond medical problems into other causes of chronic fatigue. These may involve work, relationships, personal habits, and spiritual problems.

The tired person may then continue to struggle through one day after another, perhaps stumbling onto a solution or, more likely, settling into a routine of trying to cope with life. On the other hand, he or she may join the ranks of those who seek alternative help. Diet and exercise books abound, dispensing advice both sensible

17

and silly. Friends and relatives usually have a suggestion or two. A local health-food store may offer a supplement package. Practitioners with exotic treatments and dubious credentials are ready and willing to treat chronic fatigue, usually with more time and empathy than members of the medical mainstream are able to give.

This book is written for people who still may be searching for energy—especially those whose doctors have told them they are basically okay but who still don't feel any better. It's important at the outset to define this book's scope and to lay out some guidelines for its use.

Above all, *Energy Drainers, Energy Gainers* is an informal resource, not an encyclopedia. It is intended to offer an approach to your fatigue problem (or someone else's). It will not contain the last word on every possible cause of fatigue known to the human race.

This book should be a supplement to whatever advice you have been given by your own physician, who knows you better than I do. If something you read here seems to contradict what your doctor has told you, discuss it with him or her. (I don't particularly appreciate it when the advice I have carefully spelled out to a patient is brushed aside in favor of the latest wisdom from newsstand magazines or a well-meaning but uninformed relative.)

This book contains neither quick nor surefire solutions. It is an overview of many possible energy leaks and a guide to possible ways to repair them. In addition, this book will do nothing by itself. It does not emanate healing vibrations from anointed ink. Whatever builds your energy will require your participation. Furthermore, simply *knowing* what to do isn't enough. The hassles of the real world or your personal conflicts can easily defeat the best intentions. Therefore I will frequently point out some common obstacles to making necessary changes and offer a friendly word of encouragement (or a verbal kick in the pants).

Above all, these pages have been inspired and motivated by tired people with whom I have struggled to define energy drainers and gainers. Over and over I have felt the frustration of "so many issues . . . so little time." I have also seen how chronic fatigue can cripple creativity, productivity, and joy. Furthermore, no single book has contained the perspectives I have wanted to communicate with the chronically tired. Necessity has thus become the mother of many hours at the word processor. My hope and prayer is that you will benefit from the result.

TWO
Energy and Fatigue: Some Basic Principles

Raring to go. Bursting with energy. All charged up. Full of steam.

Pooped. Shot. Exhausted. Drained. Wiped out. Out of gas. Ready to drop.

These word pictures are not exactly scientific definitions, but they vividly express the feelings conveyed by the words *energy* and *fatigue*. In order to understand these terms more clearly, however, we need to introduce some definitions and explore some specific categories.

The *American Heritage Dictionary* defines *energy* as "the capacity for action or accomplishment." Energy can be defined explicitly in physical science; chemical, electrical, or atomic energy, for instance, can be measured with appropriate tools. However, we have no way to measure human energy levels. We have only observations of what people do and their own statements about how they feel. The study of human energy and fatigue thus tends to be far more descriptive than statistical.

We tend to think of human energy in terms of

activity. Small children provide the most intense examples of this. After watching many weary mothers with young children careening off the walls of an exam room, I have often fantasized about finding a technique to transfuse energy from children to parents. It's very unusual to see chronic fatigue in a child under the age of ten in the absence of a medical problem.

This book's references to energy, especially in the context of energy drained and gained, indicate the subjective sense of well-being and the capacity for activity, as defined above. *This concept of energy relates to the totality of physical, mental, and spiritual health.* It does not relate in any way to the mystical notion of "universal life energy" (such as *Ch'i* or *prana*) that is central to many of the practices of New Age medicine. While some people who are chronically tired have been drawn to therapies based on "life energies," there are serious reasons to doubt the validity of these therapies on both scientific and biblical grounds. I have written at some length about these approaches to health care in another book, *New Age Medicine.*[1]

It's important to note that being energetic should not be considered as an ultimate goal in itself. Remember that a person can be highly energetic in criminal, immoral, or psychotic behavior as well as in constructive pursuits.

Fatigue, in obvious contrast, is "physical and mental weariness," that may be manifested by decreased activity and accomplishment. "Being tired" may refer to a transient feeling arising from one night's lost sleep, the symptom produced by a serious illness, or a chronic orientation to life. Fatigue may be *acute,* related to a specific event such as a long hike or an "all-nighter" spent completing a term paper; acute fatigue will be relieved by rest. Fatigue may also be *chronic*, lasting weeks or months on end.

Interestingly, many people who state they are chronically tired still carry out their daily routines, whether out of habit, necessity, or self-discipline. They do what needs to be done, though they feel sick while doing it. Others, especially those with overt medical illness, will be unable to carry out even their most basic responsibilities. Those who are severely depressed will be flatly apathetic about their lack of activity.

DIFFERENT TYPES OF FATIGUE

While it hardly takes a medical degree to know you're tired (and how long you've been that way), understanding why and what to do may require some investigation. Unfortunately, fatigue is only a symptom, not a diagnosis. Just as there are many kinds of headaches (muscle contraction, migraine, sinus, etc.), there also are several types of fatigue. Sometimes more than one type occurs in the same person.

Physical fatigue caused by disease. Most people who seek medical advice about fatigue are worried that a serious illness may be the underlying cause. However, in only a small percentage of tired patients is this, in fact, the case.[2] This type of fatigue may be acute (such as the malaise of a flu) or chronic (such as the draining effects of a widespread cancer) and is the type most readily identifiable by a doctor. Chapters 4, 5, and 6 will examine diseases that (do and don't) cause chronic fatigue.

Physical fatigue caused by habits and lifestyle.

This type of fatigue is far more common than that caused by actual disease. Obesity, erratic eating patterns, poor physical conditioning, disrupted sleep, as well as the effects of prescription, nonprescription, and recreational drugs are important reasons for tiredness. Unfortunately, the effects of these drugs are often difficult to overcome. Chapters 7 through 10 will explore this type of fatigue.

Acute mental and emotional fatigue. This fatigue can usually be attributed to a specific event: a difficult homework assignment, preparing income-tax returns, packing for a long trip, hosting a pack of in-laws for Christmas, and so forth. Episodes like these and the tiredness they create are usually self-limited. More serious events that are relatively brief in duration—the sudden death of a loved one, a business reversal, or a divorce—will have both immediate and long-lasting repercussions that can contribute to fatigue for months or years.

Depression. Fatigue is frequently the primary complaint of a depressed person, whether that depression is related to outside circumstances (reactive), internal biochemical processes (endogenous), or a mix of both. Depression may be acute, chronic, or recurrent. Some professionals argue that all chronic fatigue basically represents a depressive problem unless there is an obvious medical disorder; this book does not make this assumption. Nevertheless, many tired people feel considerably better after they are treated appropriately for depression. Many professionals also overlook the spiritual dimensions of fatigue-related depression. Yet a person's energy and fatigue can be profoundly influenced by moral conflict, unhealthy attitudes, and

23

the direct involvement of God (or his enemies). We'll take a closer look at these issues in chapter 11.

Chronic mental and emotional fatigue. This kind of fatigue is very frequently present in those who seek a medical evaluation. It often involves long-term conflict or dissatisfaction with relationships, job, and the circumstances of everyday life. Very often someone with this type of fatigue is fighting battles on more than one front. Verbal gunfights all day at work may be followed by a trench war at home, for example. We will review this fatigue problem in more detail in chapters 12 and 13.

BASIC PRINCIPLES ABOUT FATIGUE

People who are chronically tired have usually spent a number of waking hours (or sleepless nights) thinking about the possible causes of their problem. Many have come up with some reasonable ideas. Others remain perplexed. And a few arrive at conclusions that are farfetched or even bizarre.

In order to get a realistic perspective on the problem of chronic fatigue, we need to examine a few basic principles. While one or more of these principles may seem painfully obvious at first glance, I'm often impressed by the difficulty many tired people have grasping them. Furthermore, the principles apply to virtually all the material that follows in this book. Bear with me.

Fatigue Is Subjective

Fatigue, like pain, is subjective. As noted earlier, we have no scientific units for measuring fatigue. More importantly, *fatigue is usually drastically influenced by one's current emotional state and especially by one's expectations for the immediate future.*

We need only observe our children, or recall our own childhood, to see this illustrated vividly. Watch their behavior on Christmas morning, for example. Notice how they pound on the face of anyone resembling an adult at five o'clock in the morning (a wonderful experience for those who have been up until three o'clock assembling the Batman Big Wheels and the Barbie Hot Tub). But watch them again on any Monday morning during school months. Notice how an earthquake, a fire alarm, or the Marine Corps Band fails to get their attention. Observe how they stagger to the bathroom, pull on clothes without opening their eyes, and mumble nothing particularly meaningful for at least half an hour.

On rare occasions, our family has taken off a midweek day during school in order to enjoy Disneyland without fifty thousand other people. For added fun and research for this book, we have also neglected to notify our children of our plans until the actual morning arrived. After listening to a few of their moans and groans about waking up, we casually say something like, "You need to get dressed so we can leave for Disneyland." The results are miraculous, something no medical breakthrough could ever duplicate. A few words signaling a change in the day's agenda from social studies to Star Tours trigger an amazing burst of activity.

A variation on this theme can occur in the setting of a medical problem, whether major or minor. Mild symptoms can be ignored when circumstances are enjoyable and interesting, but they become a ball and chain in the face of an unpleasant task. School-age children are notorious for complaining on Monday morning about a cold that they ignored on Saturday. Our son Chad once survived a hot summer day of whirling and churning rides at a local amusement park while he was fighting a stomach flu. His endurance of this expensive abuse was nothing short of amazing. But in September, a trip to school under the same circumstances would have been out of the question.

This tendency to override or fixate on symptoms will vary from person to person and time to time, but it is particularly important with fatigue, which impacts on every activity of the day. It also should be noted that this process is not the same as the age-old art of goldbricking, the deliberate faking of nonexistent illness in order to be excused from some unpleasantries.

Chronic Fatigue Rarely Has One Cause

Occasionally I will see a patient who has a single problem that is creating tiredness. More often, in about nine out of ten cases, fatigue is like a river that is fed by several streams. Several years of a few calories a day too many may create a twenty-pound or eighty-pound burden to carry. A job may be a constant irritation, or the daily round of chores at home may feel like an endless treadmill. A stack of bills may overwhelm the paycheck. A long-neglected relationship may have sunk to an insufferable level. Spiritual issues may underlie all of the above. And there may be a medical problem lurking behind the scenes. Defining the problems and mapping these various streams may be a major challenge, requiring some serious thinking, with or without the help of a professional. Yet identifying causes is only the beginning.

Chronic Fatigue Rarely Has a Single Cure

The person who enters the doctor's office asking for "something to pep me up" will usually be disappointed, especially if the practitioner is reputable. Alas, many fortunes have been made selling pills, potions, and shots to the weary, not to mention miracle diets, animal extracts, and electrical stimulators. More recently, with the emergence of New Age medicine under the banner of holistic health, the playing field has widened enormously to include all sorts of cures: from ancient civilizations, crystals, psychic healing, and infusions of "universal energy."

For some people these approaches seem to improve matters for a while, for reasons that make little or no sense biologically. More often, New Age practitioners do something very important: they convince tired people that there is indeed a specific cause and cure for the fatigue. The miracle diet or energy balancing or toxic cleansing works for a while, but then the fatigue tends to creep back like weeds in a garden. The industrious but still-tired person will then continue the search for something else, an elusive Holy Grail full of perpetual energy.

Chapter 5 will take a look at a few popular but questionable causes of chronic fatigue, such as hypoglycemia, candida (the yeast, not an opera), and mysterious, unidentified "toxins" that supposedly can be exorcised by rigid dietary regimes. These theories, unfortunately, cause many people to fixate on an imaginary tree while ignoring a real forest.

Treatment for Fatigue Requires Effort

Chronically tired people who are planning to plug their energy leaks need to face an irritating paradox: The treatment in most cases requires *effort* on the part of the tired person. This is especially true in situations where dietary changes and exercise programs are in order. The person who is too tired to do what will reduce tiredness is like the hero of the old song about the hole in the bucket: he couldn't fix the hole because the critical ingredient needed was water, which would run out of the hole. Unfortunately, there are few passive cures for chronic fatigue. Not many things that are done to us or for us will raise energy levels on a lasting basis.

Increasing Energy Is a Slow Process

It should come as no surprise that raising energy levels is usually a slow process. Most chronically tired people can't say exactly when their weariness started, and few can identify exactly when things began to improve. Managing chronic fatigue is like steering an ocean liner: a number of small course corrections will result in a change in position some time later.

Chronic Fatigue May Need Medical Evaluation

In general, significant fatigue lasting more than two weeks should be evaluated medically, unless there is an obvious cause, such as lack of sleep caused by a fussy newborn. Even though specific medical treatment may not be needed, and even though the poking, prodding, and expense will most often lead to the famous conclusion, "I don't see much wrong with you," tiredness may be the result of a serious problem that needs immediate attention or a simpler one with a straightforward solution.

Two cases from my own experience illustrate this. The car painter mentioned in chapter 1 turned out to be severely anemic—that is, he had about one-third of the normal number of red cells in circulation. After thoroughly examining him, we discovered an iron-deficiency anemia caused by an extremely poor diet. His daily beer consumption was displacing calories he needed to get from more useful food. Some iron supplementation, a serious discussion about eating habits, and a decision to send Spuds McKenzie to the dog pound improved his energy levels within several days.

A woman in her early fifties came into my office unable to understand why she had been so worn out for the past three months. She was also unusually jumpy and had lost several pounds without any specific effort. A simple lab panel showed that her thyroid gland was cranking out an excessive amount of hormone. Her metabolism was causing her to feel like a car idling too fast. Specific treatment both lowered the thyroid hormone level and markedly improved her energy level.

How can you get some initial clues about the causes of chronic fatigue? In the following chapter we will look at several key questions that can help steer you in the right direction.

THREE
A Questionnaire

Patients have often approached me as if I were a fortune-teller at the county fair. When questions about headache, back pain, or fatigue spill out one after the other with the expectation that my answers will pop back in a flash, I feel tempted to don a turban, place the medical chart against my forehead, and utter the first words that enter my mind. Most medical practice, unfortunately, is not like playing The Great Carnac, M.D., but is much more like detective work—methodical, persistent, and at times tedious. A lot of questions need to be asked, and a lot of leads may need to be pursued, including some that draw blanks. In addition, a lot of thinking and temporizing (the medical term for "Let's wait and see what happens") are often in order, especially with some of the tougher problems such as chronic fatigue.

Here, at no extra charge, we will walk together through a sequence of questions that help pin down causes of tiredness. Following each set of questions are some comments about a number of possible answers.

A Questionnaire

Obviously, this is no substitute for a formal medical history taken by a professional. It is impossible to produce a cookbook approach that realistically assesses all of the past experiences, heredity, personality, current circumstances, and physical condition of any person. Indeed, grandiose predictions about "computer M.D.s" are woefully naive. Only another human being, or God, can begin to size up a person in all of his or her dimensions.

Age

How old are you? The age of the tired person will suggest specific reasons for fatigue. As mentioned earlier, a chronically fatigued child under the age of ten often has a medical problem. If he or she complains of tiredness only at certain times, such as immediately before school, this suggests a different issue. The smaller the child, the more worrisome lethargy becomes as a sign of disease.

In an adolescent, chronic fatigue far more commonly represents the convergence of several streams: rapid growth, hormonal changes, erratic or bizarre eating habits (including overt eating disorders), increasingly difficult schoolwork, concerns over relationships to peers and parents, and extremely demanding schedules. I have talked to teenagers whose weekly calendar of activities—classes, job, sports, church, music, and so on—make a corporate president look like a couch potato.

One illness that is notorious for causing teenagers to be fatigued for weeks is infectious mononucleosis, whose name refers to the striking presence of particular types of white cells in the bloodstream. This disease usually produces fever, sore throat, and swollen lymph nodes in the neck, accompanied and then followed by profound weariness. Occasionally fatigue is the primary symptom, without the other frills. (By the way, mononucleosis is not spread primarily by kissing, as the venerable high-school legends have claimed.) Mononucleosis represents an unpleasant encounter with a common organism called the Epstein-Barr virus, which recently was presumed to be the cause of chronic fatigue in adults. (This is most likely not the case, as we will see in chapter 6.)

In young and midlife adults, the causes of chronic fatigue run the gamut from physical disease to spiritual conflict, usually with a variety of factors other than disease playing a role in the problem. In elderly people, physical ailments are much more likely to enter the tiredness equation, but unhealthy attitudes also can be major energy drainers.

Onset

How long have you been tired? Did your fatigue problem begin suddenly or gradually? Often the answers to these questions are vague: "I can't remember when it started," or "I've been tired for years." In general, fatigue that has snuck up on someone and then persisted for months on end is not likely to be caused by a specific disease. In contrast, when people say they became tired recently (within the past six months) or when they can state specifically when the trouble started ("I felt great until June 15"), a medical problem is more likely.

A Questionnaire

Sometimes when the time frame is uncertain, it helps to consider when you last felt really well. If the answer is, "Well, really never," your life is probably loaded with energy drainers that need plugging.

Limitation of Activities

Does the fatigue interfere with any daily activities? Have you canceled any plans because of fatigue? As noted in the first chapter, many people *feel* tired even while they are very active and productive. In fact, their fatigue may be related to overcommitment. Some, however, are so profoundly affected that their lives are constricted by tiredness. When work, recreation, and even the basic functions of life are disrupted, certain diagnoses need special consideration. *Medical disorders* should be carefully ruled out. Severe *depression* can lead to a vegetative state: confined to bed with windows shut and doors locked. Finally, a specific disorder now called *chronic fatigue syndrome* by the Centers for Disease Control in Atlanta is characterized by devastating fatigue that seriously curtails daily activities. This special problem is the subject of chapter 6.

Other Symptoms

Were there any other symptoms when the fatigue began? Are there specific physical symptoms accompanying the fatigue now? A wide variety of symptoms may accompany fatigue. Those that occurred at the onset of the fatigue problem or perhaps those that preceded it may provide some important clues about the cause. For example, a complex of fever, aches, loss of appetite, and headaches that are then followed by prolonged tiredness usually suggests that a virus started the problem and left fatigue in its wake.

Symptoms that accompany fatigue on a long-term basis also suggest directions to explore. Some explicitly point toward a physical disease: fever, unexplained weight loss, diarrhea, and rash or other generalized skin changes are examples of symptoms that demand further medical evaluation, even if they lead to dead ends. Symptoms such as insomnia, poor concentration, dizziness, and numbness or tingling that migrates all over the body may point to specific illness. Very often, however, these symptoms will turn out to be related to psychological conditions such as anxiety and depression. Sometimes when physical symptoms and mood problems mix, it can be difficult to determine which is the cart and which the horse. We will take a detailed look at a number of symptoms in the next chapter.

A word to the wise: Before seeing a physician about any particular symptom, try to think over some specific characteristics. How long has it been present? What, if anything, makes it better or worse? Has it ever happened before? Some symptoms (for example, dizziness) are notoriously difficult to pin down and may require some detailed questioning to sort out. If you have a number of complaints, don't be disappointed if all of them can't be addressed fully in one sitting.

Another word to the wise: Your physician will either tune out or become very discouraged by an intense "organ recital." No one can deal intelligently with symptoms spewed forth like machine-gun bullets. In addition, avoid at all costs the infamous phrase, "By the way . . ." I always appreciate a patient who walks in with a definite agenda and states the issues at the outset: "I have a sore shoulder, a wart on my finger, and some pains in my stomach." Knowing the topics ahead of time allows for efficient budgeting of time and effort. The shoulder may not need quite as much time if there are stomach aches to explore. But if "By the way . . ." ends the visit and turns out to be a serious problem that can't be put off, everyone in the waiting room will have to wait a lot longer.

Fluctuations

Is tiredness related to any particular activity? Is it relieved by a night's sleep? Does it change on weekends and during vacations? As noted earlier, human energy levels often change enormously, depending on circumstances and expectations. At times a lot of medical evaluation can be avoided by observing a tired person's response to a vacation. If fatigue disappears at five o'clock every Friday night or evaporates on the beach at Maui, chances are that work is a major energy drainer. On the other hand, if weariness interferes with or aborts an activity that would normally be relished, a medical problem or a significant depression are more likely.

The relationship of fatigue to sleep is an important one. If tiredness stems from too many irons in the fire and a shortage of hours left over in the day for sleeping, a long night of snoozing or a weekend catching up can work wonders. In this case, a serious look at the problem of overcommitment is in order. On the other hand, chronically tired people often complain that they feel no better after a full night's sleep than they did when they went to bed.

35

Why Am I So Tired All the Time?

Sleep is also an important issue for the depressed person, who almost invariably complains of chronic fatigue. A common symptom of depression is disturbed sleep—difficulty falling asleep, waking early, or a strong desire to sleep both night and day. We will take a closer look at this in subsequent chapters.

Past History

Has any problem like this happened before? If fatigue is a relentless companion through life or a recurrent theme with variations from one year to the next, energy drainers related to lifestyle, relationships, attitudes, and spiritual issues probably need some exploration. Depression, which often occurs in unpredictable cycles, should also be considered. Chronic disease that is overt (for example, highly active arthritis or disabling lung disease) will frequently produce tiredness. But in such cases the person at least knows what is causing much of the fatigue.

Medication

Are you taking any medications? Unfortunately, the tools of modern medicine may contribute dramatically to chronic fatigue. The most common offenders are drugs that lower blood pressure, antihistamines (used to treat allergy), and of course those compounds that are supposed to be sedating. Whether a given medicine is in fact the culprit, however, may be harder to prove than one might think. Furthermore, a medication that usually causes no fatigue at all in the general population may be

36

a major drainer for a particular individual. There will be more on this later.

Stress

Do you face major conflicts? Job pressures? Marital disruption? A child declaring war on the family? Moral dilemmas? A suffocating load of debt? As we have mentioned already, constant conflict and dissatisfaction are more often the cause of chronic fatigue than are medical maladies. Unfortunately, identifying these battle zones may be much easier than ending the wars.

Exercise

Are you involved in any specific exercise or sports activity? Regular exercise is one of the few, genuine energy gainers available—that is, it represents a way to build energy, not merely plug a leak. I rarely see a chronically fatigued person who is engaged in a consistent, meaningful exercise program. But how can anyone who is terribly weary get out and exercise? The good news is that there are some practical ways to get started, as we will see in chapter 7.

FOUR

I Told You
I Was Sick

Virtually everyone who is chronically tired worries at
some point about the possibility of a physical disease.
This chapter will look at some common medical causes
for chronic fatigue and in doing so will address two very
basic questions. First, what are some of the common
symptoms that accompany chronic fatigue, and what
might they mean? Second, what are the *types of disease*
that can bring fatigue with them? Once again, please
remember that this thumbnail sketch of various symptoms and diseases is not intended to be a medical
encyclopedia or to substitute for a discussion with a
professional. These are perspectives, not tablets of
stone.

SYMPTOMS THAT ACCOMPANY FATIGUE

The symptoms listed below often accompany
fatigue. A few of these always indicate that a medical
problem is at hand, some rarely do, and most require
some expertise to interpret. As we look at these symp-

toms, the distinction between *pathological* (disease-related) problems and *functional* disorders will be a recurring theme. In pathological problems, a specific abnormality in the tissue can be found. It may be grossly obvious to the naked eye or detectable only by microscopic or lab evaluation. In functional disorders, the tissues are not actually diseased, but they do not work as they should. A tough but common problem in medicine is determining whether someone's complaint falls into one or the other category. For example, cramping pains in the abdomen might be caused by colitis (inflammation of the large intestine), which can be treated medically. But they also can be caused by irritable bowel syndrome, in which a normal-appearing colon goes into painful spasmodic contractions at inopportune times. This condition responds to diet changes, medications at times, and even counseling or problem solving on the home or work front. (Both of these colon problems, by the way, may be associated with chronic fatigue.)

To make matters even more confusing, most of the symptoms listed below (except fever) can be experienced by people who are anxious and/or depressed. Someone who is chronically fearful may experience chest pressure, headaches, or cramping in the abdomen—individually or all at once. These discomforts are not imaginary. However, they may be given an inappropriate amount of mental attention for any number of reasons.

Fever over 100°F is always significant, whether it lasts one day or weeks. Chronic fatigue accompanied by a daily temperature elevation to this level means that a search for a medical problem is in order. Chronic infection, various forms of arthritic disease, and even cancer are among the possibilities. However, before getting panicky about fever, consider two things: First, simply feeling hot or sweaty does not indicate that a fever is present. Only a reliable thermometer can be trusted. Many people feel hot for reasons other than true temperature elevation. Second, a person's temperature normally changes in a daily cycle, possibly rising a degree or more at the end of the day. This fluctuation may range above 99°F, but rarely over 100°. If there is a question about possible fever, check temperatures both morning and evening for a few days.

Symptoms involving the head and neck are not unusual in tired people. Headache commonly accompanies fatigue and may be both an energy drainer or a symptom of another problem altogether. Furthermore, there are many possible causes for headache, ranging from everyday muscle-contraction discomforts (the familiar "Excedrin headache") to life-threatening disorders. If headaches are a relatively new problem, are disruptive, are getting worse, or are causing awakening from sleep, a visit to a physician is in order.

Certain headaches are more often associated with chronic fatigue. Sinus infections, for example, can create both tiredness and pressure or pain in the head. Nagging muscle-contraction headaches can be a major energy drainer, even though they don't represent a threat to life. Migraine headaches (a term that refers to a very specific type of headache pattern involving changes in the blood vessels of the head), on the other hand, are very disabling when they occur, but they do not usually cause chronic tiredness once they are over.

Nasal congestion or drainage on a chronic basis

40

usually is caused either by allergy (with watery drainage) or by bacterial infection (with goopy green or yellow drainage). Either situation may be accompanied by fatigue that should improve with proper treatment. Unfortunately, many of the antihistamines used to treat allergies can also cause tiredness (see chapter 9).

Dizziness is a difficult symptom to sort out. This catchall word can refer to a true vertigo or spinning sensation, a light-headed or faint feeling, or just about any vague sense that something isn't right above the neck. To make matters even more confusing, the cause of the dizziness may have nothing to do with chronic fatigue.

Among the various forms of dizziness, faintness is the one most likely to give a clue to the cause of fatigue. We define fainting as a brief loss of consciousness that is resolved immediately when a person lies down. Faintness occurs when the brain's supply either of glucose (blood sugar) or oxygen is temporarily cut back. Since the brain has no capacity to store glucose, which it needs in a nonstop flow, the body vigorously protects this fuel supply. If a person's blood-sugar level falls well below normal (a state known as hypoglycemia), several mechanisms gear up to drive the glucose back to acceptable levels. For this reason, loss of consciousness from low blood sugar is *very* uncommon unless one takes an excess of insulin or one of the oral medications that lower blood glucose for the treatment of diabetes.

A drop in oxygen level, on the other hand, usually results from a sudden fall in blood pressure, which can occur for any number of reasons. The brain's response—light-headedness or an overt fainting episode—forces the person to lie down, which rapidly corrects the problem. For this reason, do not force someone who feels faint to stay upright, unless you are interested in causing brain damage. *Always* allow the fainting person to lie down.

Many of the causes of unstable blood pressure also contribute to fatigue. Viral infections can cause faintness, especially when a person changes position rapidly. Pregnancy may cause a woman to feel light-headed or to pass out. Sudden changes in heart rate may cause light-headedness, usually accompanied by feelings of pounding or fluttering in the chest.

In elderly people, fainting is a more ominous symptom. Heart attack, stroke, dehydration, and reactions to medications all need to be considered, and any of these may be related to chronic fatigue.

Margaret was living in a residential-care facility for elderly citizens when staff members reported that she could not get out of bed without feeling faint. Indeed, she was too tired and weak even to use the rest room without assistance. Unfortunately, during the previous forty-eight hours she had suffered a major heart attack— that is, one of the major coronary arteries that supply blood to the heart had become blocked, resulting in the death of a large area of the heart. Like many elderly people, she had experienced no pain at all, but she was now unable to generate enough blood flow to support even the slightest amount of activity.

Finally, anemia, a shortage of red blood cells

(whose primary function is carrying oxygen in the bloodstream), can cause both fatigue and fainting, especially when the drop in red-cell count is rapid.

Symptoms involving the chest may indicate either minor or serious disease. Coughing may be the symptom of another problem causing fatigue (for example, chronic obstruction of airflow), or the cough itself may be the cause, especially if it interferes with sleep. Seek medical attention for any cough lasting more than two weeks, sooner if there is fever.

Shortness of breath is a true wild-card symptom. On one hand, it may arise from one of several disorders that prevent oxygen from completing the journey from the air to the bloodstream: narrowed or clogged airways, inflamed or damaged air sacs in the lungs, inadequate blood flow into the chest, or mechanical restrictions of the chest wall, to name a few. On the other hand, some people with chronic anxiety are burdened with a sensation that they are not moving air far enough down into the lung. As a result they will hyperventilate, huffing and puffing more deeply and rapidly than necessary. Taken to an extreme, this produces dizziness and tingling around the lips and fingers. Either type of problem can generate prolonged tiredness, but obviously the treatments for each are radically different.

Heart palpitations (or pounding of the heart) usually result from changes in heart rhythm. Single premature beats are extremely common and rarely indicate a serious disorder. People experiencing prolonged rapid or irregular heart rates may feel light-headedness or faint, and they should be evaluated. For some people, palpitations occur in the setting of chronic anxiety or even overt panic attacks, which may be a component of ongoing fatigue.

Abdominal symptoms may be associated in a variety of ways with chronic fatigue. Abdominal pain is an important complaint that should not be ignored. A review of all of the possible types and causes of abdominal discomfort is beyond the scope of this book and should be sorted out with a physician. Likewise, nausea, unexpected weight gain or loss, and changes in bowel habits need evaluation in order to distinguish disease from problems in the basic function of the intestine or even from problems in behavior.

Problems in reproductive functions may contribute to or result from chronic fatigue. Changes in menstrual patterns are significant and should be evaluated. Excessive bleeding may lead to anemia, which in turn can cause fatigue. In addition, heavy flow (whether more frequent or longer) may be caused by changes within the uterus itself or may involve the entire hormonal system. Premenstrual syndrome (PMS) often includes fatigue during a one- or two-week interval before menstruation begins. PMS is *not* necessarily the cause of tiredness throughout the entire month, but if it is disruptive enough, it can be a serious energy drainer. Menopause, when the ovaries retire and quit producing their usual quota of the hormones estrogen and progesterone, may pass without fanfare or may trigger an unpleasant mix of symptoms, including tiredness. For some women, the replacement of the missing hormones (via tablets or the newer skin patches) produces drastic improvement; for other women, additional problems need to be solved.

Decreased sexual interest may accompany chronic

fatigue, especially in people who are depressed. A disturbance in the quality of sexual intimacy within marriage also can be a significant energy drainer.

Aches and pains in muscles and joints may represent the end product of years of minor daily traumas. They also may be caused by serious underlying immune-system disorders (for example, rheumatoid arthritis) that require aggressive treatment.

Altered sensations such as numbness, tingling, burning, or increased sensitivity are some of the most challenging symptoms to pin down, partly because they involve subjective information from the person who is feeling them. They may be caused by important disorders such as diabetes, vitamin B_{12} deficiency, hyperventilation, and alcoholism, to name a few. Bizarre patterns of unusual sensation are often seen in anxious or depressed people, frequently confusing the issue even more.

Whew! Few things are as tiring as reading about dozens of symptoms. After all, Aunt Sally probably has told you all of hers several times. But if you're a real glutton for punishment, press on to the next section about specific diseases.

DISORDERS THAT MAY CAUSE FATIGUE

Several kinds of disorders may cause chronic fatigue. Indeed, many people who come to my office worried about tiredness have a specific disease they believe (or fear) may be the cause. The following observations are meant not to instill paranoia but rather to dispel misunderstandings about certain medical problems. If you're not terribly worried about one disease or another, you may skip to the next chapter.

Infections

Most acute and chronic infections produce fatigue of varying degrees. The *common cold* virus will slow down the otherwise healthy person for a week at most. Its irritating runny nose, sneezing, scratchy eyes and throat, and dry cough can be managed with rest and one or more of the nonprescription symptom relievers. If bacteria enter the picture, the symptoms, including fatigue, may last longer. *Sinus infections* produce fatigue, along with pressure or pain in the forehead or face, often with discolored drainage from the nose or down the throat. *Bronchitis*, often seen in association with sinusitis, produces an irritating cough, phlegm, and often fatigue. Both of these can be calmed down with antibiotics, which are otherwise useless in combating the many cold viruses.

Pneumonias are more serious infections involving the lung tissue itself (as opposed to the airways in bronchitis). Fever, chills, aches, and cough are typical, along with marked fatigue. During the winter months, *influenza* can create a very similar picture, often with more profound body aches.

Many common viruses produce general misery without involving the nose, throat, or chest. A combination of fever, aches (including headache), decreased appetite, and a profound affinity for bed—without other specific symptoms—is often called a "flu-like illness," even though the influenza virus is nowhere in sight. Viruses that produce such misery can be sent packing

46

only by using three basic treatments: rest, rest, and rest. This allows the immune system to do its job. Fluids, pain relievers, chicken soup, and vitamins have been recommended with variable fervor over the decades, but they do not help unless the sick person is also taking it easy. (Notice that your mother could provide this same advice.)

Of great importance in understanding pneumonias, influenza, and flu-like illnesses is the concept of *acute* and *convalescent* periods in the disease. The acute phase encompasses the most intense symptoms: fever, aches, chills, and coughs, which last anywhere from a day or two up to a few weeks. The convalescent phase is marked primarily by fatigue and may last quite a bit longer. Typically, the afflicted person will retire from the human race for the acute phase, then feel well enough to try a few activities. Horror of horrors, merely getting up and dressed, driving to the store, sitting through a class, or opening a few backlogged letters at work will lead to an intense desire to return to bed. This development can be both alarming and irritating, producing a lot of questions. How long will this last? How long before I can return to class, office, construction site, or land of the living? What can I do to get over this more quickly? How do I tell my teacher or boss or coach or spouse that I'm not really sick but I don't feel healthy either? Very simply, the vast majority of people will eventually get up to speed without any miracle drugs or megavitamins. Stamina will increase day by day, with the most physically demanding jobs or schedules taking the longest to restore to their former glory.

Three types of infections, however, are notorious for prolonged convalescent phases marked by serious fatigue: *hepatitis* in its various forms, *cytomegalovirus* (CMV), and *Epstein-Barr virus* (EBV). In hepatitis, the liver becomes inflamed, producing a variety of abnormalities in blood chemistries. Along with the standard flu-like symptoms, hepatitis typically produces a yellow coloration of the skin, known as jaundice, accompanied by darkening of the urine and discoloring of the stool (light or gray). The more common type-A hepatitis is acquired from contaminated food and is the most benign form. Type B—which can be transmitted sexually, through intravenous drug use, or in blood products—can be far more serious, and even lethal on occasion. Other forms, grouped under the catchall term "non A-non B," are still being characterized by medical researchers. These cause diseases of variable severity. Specific diagnosis is possible through blood tests and is important both in predicting the outcome and in preventing spread to family members or close contacts.

Cytomegalovirus (CMV) produces an intense flu-like illness, frequently accompanied by headache so intense that the treating physician may consider performing a lumbar puncture (or spinal tap) to rule out meningitis. This virus can produce some important problems for the newborn infant whose mother becomes infected during pregnancy.

The Epstein-Barr virus (EBV) is usually acquired in childhood, where it comes and goes as a routine illness. If one is unfortunate enough to have the first encounter with this invader after puberty, the manifestations are far more intense, producing the syndrome of acute mononucleosis (mono). The afflicted person (usually a teenager) endures fever, usually an intense tonsillitis, enlarged lymph nodes, major fatigue, and the harassment of classmates for having "kissing disease," which this in fact is not. Mononucleosis can be particularly irritating when it occurs during finals or some other demanding period, but it eventually runs its course. Acute mononucleosis is very uncommon in older adults. However, in recent years, many chronically tired adults have been convinced that they have a chronic form of EBV wreaking havoc in their bodies. While this is most likely not true, there is in fact a syndrome producing severe and relentless fatigue that probably represents an interaction between a virus (whether EBV or another is unknown), the immune system, and the brain. We will discuss this interesting disorder, chronic fatigue syndrome, in chapter 6.

Other infections, such as gastroenteritis (stomach flu), persistent diarrhea, kidney infections, or more exotic invasions (including the disastrous onslaughts seen as a result of collapse of the immune system in AIDS) are typically accompanied by fatigue, but the other symptoms caused by infection usually receive more attention. One exception—relatively rare in developed countries, but depressingly common in the Third World—is that of parasite infection. While some parasites announce their presence in no uncertain terms (such as with diarrhea), others may silently rob the unfortunate host of nutrients and energy. A chronically fatigued person who has traveled extensively, especially to primitive areas, should have the stools checked for parasites by a competent laboratory.

Heart, Lung, Kidney, and Liver Disorders

Congestive heart failure is a disorder in which the heart is unable to pump blood efficiently enough to manage some very basic demands of the body. Most commonly this occurs after a significant amount of heart muscle has been damaged by loss of blood supply from the coronary arteries. Other problems, including valve disease, rhythm disturbances, and diseases directly affecting the heart muscle cells (for example, alcoholism) can also disable the heart's responsiveness. When an unhealthy heart is confronted with increased demand—whether a need to move the body some distance, digest a large meal, fight an infection, overcome high blood pressure, or compensate for a loss of red cells—fluid will accumulate in the lungs (interfering with oxygen transfer and thus causing shortness of breath) and/or the liver (producing nausea) and legs (resulting in swelling). Profound fatigue often can accompany congestive heart failure, which in its worst form will affect a person at rest.

We might compare this condition to that of a car whose engine has lost two or three of its four cylinders. It will perform adequately for a few short errands, but when the driver wants to climb a mountain or put the pedal to the metal, it asks, "Who, me?" Most often congestive heart failure affects older adults. Fortunately, several measures (both dietary and medical) can help the heart pump more efficiently and also "take the load off," thus increasing stamina and prolonging life.

In *chronic lung disease* fatigue is virtually universal as the body's ability to acquire life-sustaining oxygen and exhale metabolic by-products becomes impaired. The most common form involves obstruction of airflow through narrowed bronchial tubes (chronic bronchitis) or damaged air sacs in the lungs themselves (emphysema), or both. Smoking is the most common underlying cause, though other factors including heredity can be involved. As with congestive heart failure, a number of measures can improve airflow and oxygen delivery, although some people ultimately need oxygen on a long-term basis.

Chronic kidney failure will produce fatigue if the condition is not treated. Fortunately, this is rarely the cause of tiredness in someone who has no known risk factors such as diabetes, abnormalities in the urinary tract, or severe high blood pressure. Kidney status can be assessed using routine blood and urine screening.

Chronic liver failure, like kidney failure, rarely sneaks up on anyone. Usually the process evolves over time as the result of gradual damage (typically caused by alcohol) or infection. Rarely will someone come to a medical office complaining only of fatigue and be found to have this problem. However, a person who is unfortunate enough to be suffering the full consequences of liver failure (especially cirrhosis) will be fatigued indeed, but with many more urgent problems.

Immune System Disorders

Disorders involving the immune system frequently are accompanied by chronic fatigue. *Allergies* represent an overzealous response of the immune system to one or more external agents, known as antigens. Reactions to pollens, dust, or other environmental agents can produce irritating nasal, eye, or respiratory symptoms that are energy drainers. Allergies to food may be more difficult to identify, but they most often generate intestinal complaints (especially diarrhea) or hives. Food allergies rarely cause chronic fatigue in the absence of other symptoms. This is an important concept because many chronically fatigued people believe that some mysterious food, additive, or toxin is responsible for their affliction. Furthermore, many forms of intolerance to food, such as the inability to digest the sugar in milk, are not allergic in origin.

Autoimmune disorders involve an inappropriate attack of the immune system on the body itself, a sort of physiologic civil war. Well-known examples are rheumatoid arthritis and lupus, but there are dozens of others. A gamut of symptoms involving any number of organ systems can occur, at times with disastrous results. Because joints are so often involved in these diseases, persistent or recurring joint pain accompanying fatigue should be investigated.

Immune-deficiency states have been traditionally the province of the subspecialist and the university medical center, but the onslaught of AIDS—Acquired Immune Deficiency Syndrome—is changing that picture permanently. AIDS is, in fact, the end stage of a long process set in motion by the human immunodeficiency virus (HIV). Acquired mainly through sexual contact, intravenous use of illegal drugs, and in a few cases via transfusion, the virus lies dormant for years before producing relentless changes in the body's ability to fight infection. While HIV-infected patients develop fatigue as the disease progresses, this is rarely an isolated symptom. People who have had more respiratory infections or flu-like illnesses than usual over a given period of time sometimes become concerned about the possibility of AIDS. Fortunately, few of these prove to have HIV disease. However, prolonged fever, sweats, and weight loss should be investigated, especially if there is a history of homosexual or bisexual activity, intravenous drug use, or sexual contact with people having such a history.

Endocrine Disorders

Endocrine disorders, those involving one or more of the body's hormones, can cause fatigue. Many tired people frequently suspect hormone disorder to be the source of their misery. In fact, this is usually *not* the case. *Diabetes,* in which blood sugar (glucose) is abnormally elevated, usually does not cause fatigue until some significant metabolic problems are under way. Many people live with moderately high blood-glucose levels and have no idea anything is wrong until some other complications develop. Extremely high levels, however, create a physiologic chain reaction that involves excessive urine output, thirst, weight loss, and fatigue. In some people, especially young diabetics, this can progress into a combination of life-threatening disturbances. *Hypoglycemia* (low blood sugar) is virtually never the cause of chronic fatigue, a conclusion we will discuss in the next chapter.

Thyroid disease, whether causing low levels of thyroid hormone (hypothyroidism) or the opposite (hyperthyroidism) can produce significant fatigue, but with a constellation of other symptoms. Hypothyroid patients are like a car on low idle. They typically feel sluggish, constantly cold, with voices dropping into a lower range. In some cases they may develop a form of puffiness (visible especially in the legs and face) that is not like typical fluid retention. Hyperthyroid patients are just the opposite: tremulous, hearts pounding, constantly hot, they appear "revved up" and may appear to have chronic anxiety. Both of these are easy to diagnose with routine blood tests.

As we mentioned earlier, *changing patterns in estrogen and progesterone* in women can produce a variety of symptoms and certainly contribute to fatigue. Nevertheless, sorting out exactly what is going on (other than diagnosing menopause when it occurs) may be a tricky business. The problem stems not only from the marked variations in blood levels of these hormones during the course of the month, or from month to month, but also from the high cost of measuring them.

Although some practitioners use progesterone to treat premenstrual syndrome (PMS), for example, it is extremely difficult to predict who will improve or who will worsen. Indeed, the exact hormonal picture that leads to PMS is not particularly clear. Similarly, many women with chronic fatigue believe that they have a hormone imbalance that some combination of vitamins, food supplements, shots, or suppositories can cure. Like any other single-minded quest for a miraculous fount of energy, the search for hormonal balance can be a difficult one indeed.

Susan had been seen several times over the years for significant bouts of fatigue, mood swings, and anxiety that had not responded to repeated medical evaluations (all normal) and reassurance. Hearing a radio ad for a clinic that specialized in the treatment of premenstrual syndrome, she made a crosstown drive to find out if this might be her problem. She was told that she would benefit from a rigorous regime of both estrogen and progesterone supplements, and she did indeed feel somewhat better after this plan was started. But many of the same symptoms continued to bother her, leading to self-medication with higher doses of hormone supplements.

Later she came to our office, requesting refills of her high-dose hormonal regime. Discussions at some length revealed that her symptoms were not limited to the days before her menstrual period but had extended throughout the month. Nevertheless, she persisted in her conviction that hormone imbalances alone were the cause of her various symptoms. Finally, she agreed to reduce the dosage of her supplements. Her symptoms changed very little. Eventually, more specific treatment of depression led to stabilization of her mood swings.

On the other side of the hormonal coin, some straightforward therapy can greatly improve a woman's well-being in certain situations. Replacing estrogen can help many postmenopausal women, as noted earlier. Women who are irritable, bloated, and fatigued (among other things) for one or two weeks before each menstrual period can indeed be helped in a number of ways. Simply being reassured that the bad feelings have a physical basis rather than a psychological one can help immensely. Dietary measures—avoiding salt and sugar and eating small amounts of food more frequently—are beneficial. Diuretics remove a number of pounds of retained fluid, which may actually be the cause of much of the recurrent irritability. And for some women, progesterone supplements seem to be very effective.

Other Conditions That May Cause Fatigue

Fatigue following major surgery is very common, but it often comes as a rude surprise to the adult who expects to be charging back into the daily routine shortly after an operation. This is especially true for the woman who has had a Caesarean section; the combination of a major procedure (often the culmination of a prolonged labor), blood loss, hormonal changes, and a new baby who sounds off throughout the night can produce significant fatigue for weeks after delivery.

Cancer is probably the most common concern of the chronically tired patient. Indeed, the specter of a terrible battle with cells multiplying wildly throughout the body may in itself be a significant energy drainer. Many fatigued people who learn there is no evidence of a malignant tumor lurking somewhere in their body will have a sudden surge of energy arising from their relief.

While cancers certainly can produce fatigue, especially when they are widespread, usually some additional symptoms will be present as well, depending on the type of tumor involved. Chronic localized pain, weight loss, or the discovery of an actual mass are typical complaints. Interestingly, the person who has a known cancer does not always have to battle with fatigue. With proper treatment most tumors can be controlled and some can be cured. In addition, energy drainers other than a cancer may be involved in a particular fatigue problem.

Physiologic disorders, as we noted earlier in this

chapter, create a variety of symptoms without actually causing any particular damage. Fatigue associated with these is probably not a direct part of the process but a by-product of all the ongoing aggravation. *Irritable bowel syndrome* is a very common cause of repeated and troublesome episodes of cramping pain, loose stools, and/or constipation. *Headaches,* whether caused by muscle contraction or sudden changes in blood vessels, are major energy drainers. Chronic *pains in muscles and related soft tissues* can be terribly annoying even when there is no obvious pathology (such as inflammation) in progress. Obviously, some professional input is necessary to determine whether a person has a nagging physiologic problem that needs to be controlled or a pathological one that needs specific treatment to prevent further damage.

Finally, *medications,* both prescribed and over-the-counter, can contribute to fatigue, or be the primary cause. We will review some of the major offenders in chapter 9.

FIVE

Misunderstandings About Causes of Fatigue

In recent years, hypoglycemia, chronic candidiasis, toxins, and food allergies have been targeted as common causes for chronic fatigue. In some cases these diagnoses have been marketed to the general public without any clear professional consensus as to their validity, and at times in the face of widespread criticism from experts. Unfortunately, significant sums of money have been paid to people who specialize in these diagnoses.

HYPOGLYCEMIA

Hypoglycemia, or low blood sugar, was a particularly popular diagnosis in the 1970s, and many people still wonder whether it is the cause of their fatigue. Hypoglycemia *does* indeed exist, but it is relatively rare or at least very difficult to demonstrate among those who believe they have it. The most common instances actually involve excessive intake of medications that reduce blood glucose in diabetics—insulin, which is injected, or oral agents used to assist those who do not need insulin but lack adequate control with diet alone. Serious reductions in blood sugar from insulin can lead to so-called "insulin shock," a potentially disastrous complication. Dangerous lowering of glucose from oral medicines is less common but can occur, especially in elderly people. Improvement is usually dramatic following the intake of juice or other high-carbohydrate food or after injection of glucose by vein in more extreme cases.

Many tired people who are not diabetic have been put on elaborate dietary and supplement regimes based on the assumption that their blood sugar was chronically low. In fact, random testing of glucose (or even checking when patients feel ill) virtually never demonstrates low blood sugar. Why? Because the body zealously guards against it. As we mentioned earlier, only one hormone (insulin) can lower glucose, while a number of others raise it, a safeguard against loss of fuel for the brain.

Some people complain that they feel ill after eating sweet foods, and thus they suspect that sugar in their diet is the cause of their tiredness. (Entire books are based on this premise.) In fact, a few of these people actually have *reactive hypoglycemia*, which involves an excessive output of insulin in response to a large meal or intake of sweets.[1] Other people probably have a less severe but still irritating response to such foods. Very rarely, a glucose-tolerance test (in which blood sugar is measured several times after a specified load of glucose is given by mouth) may demonstrate this process. Unfortunately, more often than not the results are not terribly illuminating because the test does not accurately duplicate anyone's normal food and activity levels.

The best course of action for anyone concerned about swings in blood-sugar levels is a simple dietary change. If you feel ill after eating sweet foods, don't eat them. To avoid swings in blood glucose, keep the intake of fuel more constant through the course of the day. For example, half of a normal lunch can be eaten at noon and the other half three hours later. Typical mealtimes are social customs based on the activity and hunger patterns of the majority of people, but they do not work for everyone. Eat a diet rich in complex carbohydrates— fruits, vegetables, and grains such as cereals, bread, rice, and pasta. These release fuel into the body slowly and should be the mainstay of such a diet (or for that matter, diets in general). I mention this because the long-discredited notion that carbohydrates are fattening is still alive and well.

CHRONIC CANDIDIASIS

Chronic candidiasis, or candidiasis hypersensitivity syndrome, is another popular explanation for chronic fatigue, but one that lacks much credibility at this time. The yeast species *Candida albicans* is no stranger to the human body. It thrives in wet and warm places: skin folds (especially in overweight people and in babies' diaper area), the vagina, and occasionally the mouth (where infection is called thrush). It is particularly fond of diabetics who are out of control (that is, with high blood sugars) and people who have been on prolonged or intensive courses of antibiotics. These infections with candida produce local irritation and itching, at times intense, and usually respond to appropriate medications applied directly to the area involved. In a small number of unfortunate people with immune deficiencies (AIDS patients or cancer patients receiving chemotherapy), candida can spread throughout the body, causing a devastating illness.

The so-called candida hypersensitivity syndrome has been described by Dr. William Crook in his book *The Yeast Connection: A Medical Breakthrough,* and subsequently has found receptive ears from coast to coast.[2] Dr. Crook's thesis is that excessive growth of *Candida albicans* in the body progresses into weakening of the immune system and thus leads to innumerable symptoms: fatigue, depression, hyperactivity, headaches, abdominal ailments, respiratory disease— the list encompasses nearly every organ system and a huge array of possible complaints. Diagnosis is based not on any particular test, or even on cultures of candida, but rather "is suspected from the patient's history and confirmed by his response to treatment."[3] Treatment encompasses a variety of approaches, including a special diet designed to limit simple carbohydrates and avoid refined foods and "all yeast and mold containing foods," which are said to encourage the growth of candida. Nutritional supplements, use of antifungal medications, and even immunotherapy in the form of injections of candida extracts are used by some practitioners.

Unfortunately, the yeast-connection theory bears all of the hallmarks of a non-disease. The person's symptoms are so vague and numerous that nearly everyone can identify at least one or two at any given time. No meaningful diagnostic tests are available other than response to a patchwork quilt of therapies. No meaningful proof suggests that *Candida albicans* can produce such generalized misery or that the proposed treatments (other than the antifungal agents) have any impact on the organism at all. I could just as easily substitute another potential biological offender—one of the common skin bacteria or house dust or cosmic rays—into this formula, publish a book for general consumption, claim that the mainstream of medicine has missed the boat, and create a loyal following (and some extra income) for years to come.

The bottom line is this: The promoters of candida hypersensitivity syndrome will need to find more convincing evidence in the coming years to support their claim that this common yeast is a cause of chronic fatigue—or anything else.

TOXINS AND FOOD ALLERGIES

Toxins and *food allergies*, terms that have a specific meaning in mainstream medicine, are used widely in yet another dubious approach to chronic fatigue and other health problems. Material published in books, pamphlets, and newsletters originating from a distinct nutritional subculture claims that innumerable disorders are caused by accumulations of toxins in the body, most of which are said to arise from modern methods of food preparation. Consider the following example:

> When we eat foods that are cooked, processed, white flours-refined, adding to that additives, chemicals, preservatives, pesticides, sugars, etc., there is little to give the body the nutrients it needs to operate efficiently. When we have insufficient vitamins and minerals in our diet, our enzymes (the

spark of life) break down. We can no longer digest
even the foods that we are eating. This leaves
undigested TOXIC WASTE. The body circulates
this back to the toxic dump (the liver) for detox-
ification. After years of abuse it has a full station
and must send it off into the body. This then
creates the well-known histamine response.[4]

The accumulated toxins are said to provoke an
allergic response, manifested by an enormous variety of
symptoms. Not only are familiar allergic problems such
as runny nose and asthma mentioned, but other more
unusual disorders are included as well: epilepsy,
speech problems, autism, obesity and inadequate
weight, constipation and diarrhea, abnormal body odor,
hemorrhoids, bedwetting, and vaguely defined "heart
problems" and "bladder problems."

Testing for food allergies and toxins problems is
carried out in a variety of ways, none of which is
accepted within the scientific community as valid in this
context. *Hair analysis* is frequently promoted. While
legitimately used in certain toxicology studies (particularly in the detection of heavy metals such as mercury
and lead), it has been widely criticized as too unreliable
to serve as a routine test of nutritional status. *Cytotoxic
testing* involves the mixing of white cells with food
extracts, with the assumption that a reaction on the part
of the cell indicates allergy to the food. This concept,
while intriguing in theory, is used neither in immunol-
ogy research nor in any standard reference laboratory.
Electroacupuncture testing reportedly "checks the
energy of the food to compare it, if it is compatible with
the energy of the body."[5] This concept, unfortunately, is

drawn directly from the Taoist mystical concept that invisible energy (*Ch'i*) flowing through the body (and all else in the universe) plays a vital role in health and illness.

Treatment of food allergies and toxic accumulations emphasizes two fundamental approaches. First, elaborate and at times obsessive concern with foods and supplements dominates the treatment. The diet is to be purged of sugar, caffeine, red meats, processed foods, white flour, preservatives, and additives. Organic foods (those grown without chemical fertilizers or pesticides) are favored. Combining or not combining certain foods (for example, not eating protein and carbohydrate at the same meal) is said to improve digestion. Large doses of vitamins, minerals, and other supplements (e.g., bee pollen, wheat grass, barley green, etc.) are said to be extremely helpful, if not completely necessary, for good health.

Second, ongoing colon cleansing, using a variety of substances including charcoal, herbal laxatives, and in some circles enemas, is said to be necessary to rid the body of accumulated toxins. A preoccupation with the colon is pervasive in toxin and food-allergy materials, though in standard medical journals this organ is widely held to play a much less critical role in the processing of foreign substances.

While this book will not discuss all the elements of the food-allergy and toxic-accumulation subculture, we do want to point out a few weaknesses of this school of thought. First, the toxins so commonly mentioned are never specifically named. Their identification is usually based on long symptom lists, and their disappearance is based on subjective improvement. Overall, toxicology is a complex and detailed specialty within medicine, but it bears little resemblance to the vague writings of the toxic-accumulation perspective. Similarly, the basis for emphasizing the colon as the primary detoxifying organ lacks sufficient medical support. The biochemical processing of foreign substances by the liver and kidney is far more critical than the eventual exit via the intestinal tract, except in some cases of acute poisoning or overdose.

Second, while the toxins are poorly delineated, the allergic reactions are defined in excess. Allergies are, in fact, unique responses brought about by specific immunologic mechanisms in the body. Yet this perspective invokes allergies as the cause of virtually every pathological process, a theory that is too simplistic to be taken seriously. Furthermore, vague references to entire arenas of disease (e.g., bladder problems or heart disorders) are all too common in the food-allergy subculture.

Third, the concept that all of us are in desperate need of numerous vitamin, mineral, herbal, and trace-element supplements lacks reasonable documentation and defies logic. At the present time we are blessed with the greatest abundance and variety of foods in the history of the planet, and yet we are still told that the magical ingredients somehow elude us. Is the human body so poorly designed that when it is given food in adequate quantity and diversity, it still can't remain healthy? Food combining represents another lapse in common sense. How could it be that the human species has managed to survive for so long without someone discovering which foods we should or should not eat at the same time?

Why Am I So Tired All the Time?

The toxin theory claims, of course, that foods we buy today are inferior to those grown in the "good old days" (before chemical fertilizers and pesticides) and that they are hopelessly deficient in nutritional value. But in the "good old days" the food supply was erratic and unpredictable, and overt malnutrition was the rule rather than the exception. If anything, modern Western civilization suffers from overnutrition—that is, too many calories (a problem that food-allergy diets do help solve in many cases because of their emphasis on low-fat and low-sugar foods).

Finally, the emphasis on organic foods, which are said to be superior to those available at the local supermarket, raises economic as well as scientific issues. The purchasing of specially prepared and priced foods from the health-food store can be an expensive proposition, and the addition of an array of supplements can make an unhealthy dent in the budget. In many households this added expenditure might more wisely be spent on basic food purchases. Indeed, money spent on fresh, raw food products that are prepared at home will go much farther than money spent either on prepackaged frozen entrees from the supermarket or on exotic products from the health-food store.

Some people may argue that objections such as those listed above represent the disgruntled fumings of the medical establishment, which would rather push drugs than help people become healthier through natural means. Such is not the case. (Indeed, one could just as easily argue that practitioners in the food allergy and toxin subculture are primarily interested in selling supplements to people who really don't need them.) Appropriate and prudent dietary changes would, of course, eliminate a considerable amount of pathology in our society. Indeed, many of the recommendations for preventing "toxic accumulation" are very sensible: decreasing sugar and salt, reducing or eliminating caffeine and alcohol, cutting out the high-fat and high-cholesterol foods, and emphasizing substances high in fiber.

Many people who follow such guidelines could reasonably be expected to feel more energetic. But the increased energy occurs in a context of excessive and erroneous preoccupation with food and supposed toxins. No one benefits when gross misunderstanding of physiologic and disease processes are widespread. (Nutrition resources that are more scientifically accurate in their approach will be reviewed in later chapters.)

Before departing from this chapter, I would like to mention one very real and important diagnosis that, contrary to the opinion of some, does not directly cause fatigue. *High blood pressure* (also called hypertension, a word that has nothing to do with the mental state of the person involved) is a very common problem that can contribute to a number of serious complications, including stroke, kidney failure, and heart disease, if it is not adequately treated.

Unfortunately, this problem is completely silent except in its most extreme cases. Nevertheless, some people believe they can tell when their blood pressure is elevated. I have spoken with others who wonder if their chronic fatigue is caused by hypertension. In a nutshell, symptoms are completely unreliable as an indicator of high blood pressure. In fact, management of hypertension with medication is complicated by the fact that many people feel worse when they are treated. In general, fatigue may be caused by some of the *complications* of high blood pressure, but not by the pressure itself.

SIX

The Special Problem of Chronic Fatigue Syndrome

Up to this point we have described chronic fatigue as a common problem that can be caused by any of several medical disorders or by several forces at work in the same person. However, one specific form of chronic fatigue warrants a closer look: chronic fatigue syndrome (CFS). This is not a generic diagnosis, but a unique disorder in which the fatigue has a capital F. One patient, concerned that the name of the illness would trivialize the reality of the fatigue says, "Our fatigue is to ordinary tiredness what lightning is to a spark."

HISTORY OF CHRONIC FATIGUE SYNDROME

In 1984, in the resort community of Incline Village, Nevada (near Lake Tahoe), internists Paul Cheney and Daniel Peterson noted an unusual influx of patients complaining of profound fatigue, often but not always accompanied by low-grade fever, sore throat, swollen lymph nodes, and a variety of psychological disturbances. The subsequent physical examinations were not particularly impressive, laboratory studies were usually normal, and various attempts at straightforward treatment were unsuccessful. Most significantly, the patients had previously been in excellent health and did not seem to be candidates for depression or other psychological disorders that might cause fatigue.

The Incline Village epidemic became a national news item, and by 1985, medical journals began reporting this and other similar clusters of severe fatigue cases. This illness in many ways reminded clinicians of infectious mononucleosis, and the blood of some patients had carried unusually high antibodies against the Epstein-Barr virus (EBV), which causes mononucleosis. The media thus spread the word that the Incline Village outbreak and others like it were none other than a "chronic Epstein-Barr virus syndrome." In a way, this sounded plausible, since EBV is a member of the herpes virus family, whose members are notorious for living permanently but usually dormant in the people they infect. If the lowly chickenpox virus (varicella) can reactivate and cause shingles, could the equally common EBV come to life in some people and wreak havoc in its own way?

Before long, tired patients all over the country were asking for blood tests for EBV antibodies; the diagnosis of chronic Epstein-Barr virus syndrome was made left and right; and because there appeared to be no cure at hand, a cadre of EBV "specialists" with unique treatment ideas began separating a lot of tired people from their hard-earned money. Meanwhile, rank-and-file physicians began to notice that virtually *everyone* checked for EBV antibodies had them. Furthermore, more careful studies revealed that the antibody patterns of people diagnosed as having chronic EBV syndrome were also present in many people who felt perfectly well.[1] Thus the entire diagnosis became suspect and the illness was given titles like "yuppie flu" and "affluenza," since many cases involved professional young adults. Was this not simply another variation on the same old theme of tired people looking for a scapegoat disease rather than working on their own energy drainers?

DEFINITION OF CHRONIC FATIGUE SYNDROME

In many cases, this was true. People who needed to deal with depression, work on disordered relationships, or change their lifestyle became fixated on the Epstein-Barr virus, and they remained tired. But other case histories were so striking that they warranted clarification and further research. Finally in 1988, the Centers for Disease Control (CDC) published what it called a working case definition of chronic fatigue syndrome.[2] While acknowledging that the cause of CFS is unknown (and most likely not the EBV), the CDC listed a number of criteria for identifying a case as CFS. Since at this point no proven effective cure exists (though a number of coping strategies are available, many of which are encompassed in the following chapters of this book), the CDC criteria serve mainly to define cases for research purposes. In addition, the criteria help point patients and their physicians in the right direction.

The first major criterion relates to the severity of the fatigue problem. To be diagnosed as having CFS, someone must have an onset of persistent or relapsing fatigue without a previous history of similar symptoms and without improvement with bed rest. The fatigue must be severe enough to reduce daily activities by 50 percent or more for at least six months. This profound and intense fatigue, more devastating than normally seen in a typical tired patient (and in some cases more like that of the terminally ill), is the hallmark of the disorder. Patients with CFS do not simply go about their daily business feeling less energetic than usual. They become truly disabled by their fatigue, at times capable of only the most basic tasks of self-care, such as taking a shower, before returning to bed.

One person with CFS described the problems posed even by everyday activities as follows:

> I hire people to do strenuous household work—cleaning, laundry in the basement laundry room, shopping, doing errands. I have to spend energy planning how not to overexert, which for me may be not going up and down steps in our two-story house, not going to the post office, most weeks no going out except to church. I've had to learn to do most things from a reclining position. If I've had a particularly good day, my husband and I try some slow walking at night; but most nights I feel too sick even to consider it.

The second major criterion is equally important. Other medical and behavioral conditions that can produce fatigue must be ruled out by appropriate examination and laboratory studies. The CDC's list of disorders to consider is lengthy, encompassing all arenas of physical disease, many psychiatric conditions, as well as alcohol and substance abuse. (Nearly all of these are reviewed to some extent in this book.)

In addition, the CDC lists a number of minor criteria: symptoms and physical findings that must have begun at or after the onset of fatigue and that persisted or recurred for at least six months. In order to qualify as a case of CFS, a person must have eight of the following:

1. Mild fever or chills
2. Sore throat
3. Painful lymph nodes in the neck or armpit areas, less than about an inch in size (larger lymph nodes suggest other diseases)
4. Unexplained, generalized muscle weakness
5. Muscles aches (myalgias)
6. Prolonged fatigue (more than 24 hours) following exercise that would have been tolerated easily prior to the onset of illness
7. Generalized headaches (differing in pattern or severity from any experienced prior to the illness)
8. Aching joints, in various locations, without actual redness or swelling
9. Any of a number of neurological or psychological complaints, especially depression, difficulty concentrating, forgetfulness, and irritability
10. Sleep disturbances: insomnia or hypersomnia (excessive sleep)
11. Development of the main complex of symptoms over a few hours or days[3]

Researchers have noted some specific trends in CFS cases. Overall, only 3% to 5% of people who state that chronic fatigue is a major complaint fit the CDC criteria for CFS. Females with CFS outnumber males about three to one, with a typical onset in the mid-30s. In addition, most cases begin with a sudden appearance of symptoms rather than the gradual or vague development of fatigue seen in so many chronically tired patients.[4]

CAUSE OF CHRONIC FATIGUE SYNDROME

The cause of CFS remains unknown, but a number of theories are under consideration. The disorder probably will not turn out to be the work of one particular virus (as AIDS proved to be) or a single environmental agent. One of the more likely explanations is that CFS represents a subtle and complex alteration of immune function—not a devastating breakdown as occurs in AIDS, but a combination of hyperactivity and mild deficiency. The trigger for this process could be any number of viruses or perhaps a mixture of infectious and environmental agents. Indeed, the likelihood that a malfunction of the immune system is involved has led many to refer to CFS as chronic fatigue and immune dysfunction syndrome or CFIDS. Much research remains to be done, and undoubtedly the next few years will see some significant clarification of this process and its causes.

TREATMENT FOR CHRONIC FATIGUE SYNDROME

If CFS for now is defined mostly by its disruptive symptoms, with causes and treatments still up in the air, what can be done about it? The most important first step, as the CDC definition so clearly implies, is to *make sure something else is not the cause of your fatigue*. Many people have jumped to the conclusion that they have CFS (or its previous identity, chronic EBV syndrome) without an adequate evaluation for other problems. Finding a physician who is willing to listen and consider the problem carefully is of critical importance. As noted in the first chapter of this book, doctors often cringe when a chronic-fatigue problem comes through the door, since they anticipate spending a lot of time with marginal results or they may have preconceived opinions about the cause of CFS (usually that it represents depression). Many physicians are not aware that the CDC has come up with case-definition criteria for CFS, which at least gives them something into which to sink their medical teeth. Ideally, a family physician or internist will look into the problem thoroughly and then give prudent guidance over the long term, suggesting coping strategies, referring to specialists when appropriate, and listening as symptoms change.

Beyond identification of the syndrome, what else can be done? Several of the energy-gainer approaches described in the next chapters apply as much to CFS as to fatigue generated by other problems: appropriate exercise (when possible), prudent diet, stress management, dealing with daily aggravations, and so on. Medications for the most part are useful only for symptom relief: acetaminophen (Tylenol) or ibuprofen (Advil or Medipren, for example) for aches and pains, and very cautious, short-term use of sleeping agents for insomnia, if absolutely necessary, are the main examples.

Some patients have responded well to very low doses of antidepressant medications. The reasons for this are still unclear. The dosage that helps CFS patients (for example, 10 milligrams per day of Sinequan) is much too low to deal with a depression, even though depression frequently produces fatigue and even though many people who are terribly fatigued eventually become depressed.

One of the most hazardous aspects of this type of problem is the vulnerability of its victims to fringe therapies and outright quackery. After all, if mainstream medicine doesn't have much to offer, what harm could there be in a little reflexology or homeopathy? Maybe the yeast connection (chronic candidiasis) is the problem. The need to find *something* that works can be so powerful as to throw caution and reason to the wind. At the risk of sounding overly conservative, I would strongly recommend staying somewhere within the confines of the scientific mainstream and away from the New Age therapies (which have their own consciousness-changing agenda), the extremely detailed dietary treatments, the intravenous vitamins, and the exotic supplements with exotic names and more exotic price tags. This can be tricky, because some of the materials written about CFS (even the better materials) advocate unorthodox or frontier therapy. (For example, one widely distributed book entitled *Chronic Fatigue Syndrome: The Hidden Epidemic* explains and endorses a variety of New Age concepts as tools for dealing with CFS.[5]) If at all possible, discuss any proposed treatments with a primary-care physician who knows you and something about this syndrome as well.

Most CFS patients need lots of support, but unfortunately the mixture of profound symptoms and an unclear diagnosis usually begins to wear thin with family members and even with health-care providers. As a result, scores of local self-help groups have formed, usually related to one of three national organizations.[6] As with any difficult medical problem, people with CFS can benefit from the support of others who have "been there" and who may have some practical ideas for coping over the long run. On the other hand, it is very important not to become a "career" CFS patient, whose entire life is defined by illness.

Probably the most useful book about CFS is Karyn Feiden's *Hope and Help for Chronic Fatigue Syndrome: The Official Book of the CFS/CFIDS Network,* which has been written in conjunction with the three most prominent national organizations.[7] The approach in Ms. Feiden's book is multidimensional, offering perspectives both from patients and physicians who have experienced and studied this syndrome. In general, speculation about cause and advice on treatment is offered with appropriate caution, although fringe therapies such as the chronic candidiasis syndrome are given a measure of credibility. The book's list of resources, including organizations, medical journal articles, and other resources is extensive.

Another helpful book is *Chronic Fatigue Syndrome: A Victim's Guide to Understanding, Treating and Coping with That Debilitating Illness* by Gregg Fischer (New York: Warner Books, 1989). This book covers some of the same ground, but from the more personal perspective of one who is actually coping with CFS.

As noted earlier, patients with CFS need to plug energy leaks as much as those with less intense fatigue syndromes. It is now time to move ahead and consider a number of specific energy drainers and gainers.

PART II
ENERGY DRAINERS
ENERGY GAINERS

Each chapter in this section examines an energy drainer and suggests ways to combat it through a related energy gainer. Since entire books have been written about a number of these topics, and since I don't intend to re-invent the wheel, I will limit my suggestions to those that specially relate to fatigue.

For those people who already understand what they need to do, I hope that these chapters will provide encouragement and incentive to begin plugging some of your energy leaks—and to stay with it.

SEVEN

Getting Off It
and Getting On with It

Drainer—Moving muscles only when necessary
Gainer—Planned exercise with measurable progress

Now that we have explored the symptoms and possible causes of fatigue, it's time to consider how lifestyle and everyday decisions affect fatigue and energy. Without a doubt, the subject of exercise should be first on the agenda. While much of what we will cover in later chapters will help plug energy leaks, a regular exercise habit is one of the few activities that *increase* energy. I rarely see a chronically tired person who is exercising regularly and reasonably.

For some people, daily exercise is a pleasant addiction. For a few it's a fate worse than death. Most people have a vague sense that they should exercise more, but they can't or won't or don't for any number of reasons. For tired people, becoming physically conditioned is like the Impossible Dream. They feel as if they lack the energy to exercise—which is what they need to do to get the energy they lack. This chapter is dedicated to those people as an encouragement and a challenge. Since there are numerous books and videos devoted exclusively to this topic, we will not describe detailed exercise regimes but rather look at *why we should* exercise and *why we usually don't.*

WHY WE NEED EXERCISE

When God designed the human body, he had the entire scope of history in mind, not merely the late twentieth century. We are born with muscular equipment intended to propel us more or less continuously during waking hours. During the past one hundred years, however, we have worked diligently to defeat that purpose. Vehicles of every description carry us over all but the shortest distances. Elevators and escalators are far more popular than stairs. Work in the Western world has shifted from physical labor toward processing information. Not many of us tote that barge and lift that bale at work, and after arriving home, we diligently use remote controls to prevent walking a few steps to adjust our favorite sources of entertainment.

Most young children, especially toddlers, have not discovered the labor-saving devices with which we are blessed and prefer to move their bodies at a blistering pace throughout the day. But by the time these tricycle motors reach the age of double digits, far too many have become confirmed couch potatoes, choosing the flicker of the cathode ray tube over the rigors of the great outdoors. If they're not pried off the sofa on a regular basis, their life span will likely be shortened.

One of the most significant studies confirming this dire prediction was recently conducted by the Institute for Aerobics Research in Dallas, Texas. Over thirteen thousand men and women in apparent good health were grouped into five different fitness levels based on their performance on a treadmill test. Over the eight-year study period, 283 died. After accounting for various risk factors (such as weight, smoking, family history, etc.), the researchers found that the death rate was markedly higher in the least fit group. Surprisingly, the second most sedentary group did much better. Death rates improved with fitness level for the other three groups, but the differences were not as dramatic as those between the bottom two groups. Their conclusion: a very modest level of exercise—such as a brisk walk for thirty minutes a day—significantly decreases, over the long haul, one's risk of death from a variety of causes, including but not limited to heart and blood-vessel disease.

Aerobic Exercise

Before proceeding further, we need to look at the type of exercise just described. *Aerobic* literally means "using oxygen" and refers to an equilibrium between supply and demand. All tissues need oxygen on a continuous basis, and it is the job of the heart and lungs to supply it as needed. When we sleep or sit still, the heart and lungs can succeed at their mission with little obvious effort, unless there is severe disease affecting either or both. Increasing levels of activity, whether crossing a room or digging a ditch, require more oxygen, and the delivery system automatically increases its output to meet the need.

With intense exertion like sprinting as fast as we can, our muscles eventually will consume more oxygen than the heart and lungs can supply, and their biochemical functioning will become *anaerobic:* occurring *without* oxygen. Obviously this state of affairs can't last long. Waste products accumulate rapidly, producing marked fatigue and bringing the activity to an end. Even after stopping, we pant for a while, paying back the "oxygen debt" we acquired while charging ahead.

If we maintain higher levels of muscle motion for a prolonged period without building up an oxygen debt, that activity is considered aerobic. Examples of aerobic exercises are walking, jogging, cycling, swimming, aerobic dancing, and cross-country skiing. In addition, certain games can be considered aerobic: soccer, basketball, racquetball, handball, and water polo. The key elements are *continuous* activity for a *prolonged* period (at least thirty minutes) at a rate that allows the heart and lungs to maintain an adequate oxygen supply to the muscles and other tissues.

When this is done regularly (at least four times per week) on an ongoing basis, the heart and lungs become more efficient at their appointed tasks, such that endurance increases—a consequence referred to as the "training effect"—along with an overall feeling of increased energy throughout the rest of the day.[1] This has both a psychological component (the satisfaction of doing the right thing for one's body) and a physiological one, possibly related to the release of internal pain and tension relievers known as endorphins. For some people, the added expenditure of calories contributes to weight reduction, and most people see improvement in their overall muscle tone and appearance.

When I ask patients about their current exercise activities, they often mention all sorts of activities. For the record, the following are *not* considered to be forms of aerobic exercise that reliably produce a training effect:

1. The average work day. "Doc, I'm walking around all day while I'm on the job." For postal carriers and meter readers, for example, this is true, but the activity level rarely causes a prolonged increase in heart rate, unless one is being chased by a pit bull. Even people who are on their feet all day need to schedule a specific exercise time.

2. Body building. Lifting weights and fighting Nautilus machines builds up both muscles and sweat, but these usually involve short bursts of anaerobic effort. Indeed, the anatomies that grace the pages of body-building magazines are often poorly conditioned from an aerobic standpoint. Conversely, a marathon runner rarely has a "great build." There's nothing wrong with a supervised program to improve one's looks, but it should allow time for the conditioning of the heart and lungs as well.

3. Stop-and-go sports. Golf, tennis, softball, and downhill skiing are examples of wholesome and at times vigorous popular sports that nevertheless do not create the prolonged increase in oxygen consumption necessary for an aerobic training effect.[2] This is not to say that they can't be energy gainers, however. The *recreational* benefits of these activities can make them an important tool in stress management for many people.

WHY WE DON'T EXERCISE

Like many worthwhile activities, exercise is easier to talk about than to do, especially on a regular basis.

Before reviewing specific types of exercise, we need to take a hard look at some of the reasons many people never get started and why they don't stick with it consistently.

Physical Barriers

First of all certain physical conditions make aerobic exercise difficult, if not impossible. Severe infirmity (especially in elderly people) or major congenital deformities are obvious examples. All who are chronically ill or handicapped obviously should have professional input regarding the type of exercise in which they might participate.[3] Those with chronic fatigue syndrome (CFS) have a special problem—often even the mildest exertion aggravates their weariness for hours thereafter. As will be noted later, they must move at their own (often very gradual) pace.

Assuming that a person is not dealing with a major physical problem, what other medical concerns might be important? First and foremost, there should be little if any doubt about the heart's ability to handle the proposed exercise. Some people are afraid to exercise because they fear a heart attack. The specter of Jim Fixx and "Pistol Pete" Maravich comes to mind: If these well-conditioned people dropped dead while exercising, how can I be sure I won't? Actually, these two tragedies are like airline crashes—very rare and not representative of the millions who exercise regularly without a catastrophe. In Jim Fixx's case, serious warning signs of coronary artery disease were ignored because he believed, erroneously, that a highly conditioned person can't have such a problem.[4] Pete

Maravich, on the other hand, had an extremely rare and severe defect in his coronary arteries from which he should have died long before he turned forty. The fact that he played basketball vigorously and lived as long as he did was nothing short of miraculous.

Fortunately, for most people the risk of having a major problem with the heart during exercise is extremely low. Indeed, overall the risk of not exercising should provoke more fear and trembling. However, some definite precautions are important. If you are thirty-five or over, get a thorough evaluation by your physician before embarking on any significant change in activity level. This should focus specifically on risk factors for coronary artery disease—the progressive closing of the arteries that supply the heart. If these blood vessels are seriously clogged by deposits of fatty grunge, they may not be able to provide enough blood to the heart during exercise. This in turn could lead to heart-muscle damage or even a life-threatening rhythm disturbance.

Certain risk factors—age, sex, and family history—can't be changed. (Being male, over forty, and the owner of a pedigree full of people who have had heart attacks stacks the deck without anything else being wrong.) Cigarette smoking, high blood pressure, elevated blood cholesterol, and excessive weight all are *modifiable* risk factors—those over which we have some control, believe it or not.

Depending on the number and severity of risk factors, it may be appropriate to undergo a treadmill evaluation before embarking on a serious exercise program. This procedure, which can be done either in a physician's office or in a hospital's outpatient cardiology department, involves a carefully supervised but challenging time of exercise—walking at gradually increasing speed and incline—while the electrical activity of the heart is monitored for various abnormalities.[5] Just who should have a treadmill test? Dr. Kenneth Cooper, who has written extensively on this subject and who founded the Aerobics Center in Dallas, Texas, has recommended treadmill testing for any person who is over thirty-five and who intends to begin exercising. Others have suggested that the decision should rest on the number of risk factors involved and the intensity of exercise anticipated.[6]

In general, there is little to be said *against* having a treadmill test. The procedure is extremely safe when conducted by well-trained personnel, and it provides a useful indication of one's tolerance of vigorous exercise. The primary drawbacks are cost (usually around $350 or more) and the possibility of misleading results. *False positive* stress tests suggest that coronary disease is present when the arteries are in fact wide open. Here, the main problem is the cost of further testing to settle the question. On the other hand, *false negative* tests are potentially more damaging: here, one would believe he or she is fine when in fact there is some risk. Fortunately, these are less common than false positive results.

Aside from being aware of one's heart status, other potential physical problems need to be kept in mind. Exercises such as jogging (or even walking) may jostle the lower spine, hips, knees, or ankles, causing pain or even actual damage. Walking or running on a dirt, grass, or a sandy surface rather than pavement, and wearing appropriate walking or running shoes, can reduce the risk of this complication. For people who already have orthopedic problems, swimming is an excellent alternative, although it obviously requires access to a pool.

Other physical obstacles to exercise are environmental. Only the most dedicated jogger will trot through the snow or extreme heat. In some cities traffic, stray dogs, and even muggers put a serious damper on efforts to stay fit. Those who want to ski cross country—the most efficient form of aerobic exercise—need to live where the conditions and terrain are appropriate. Those who prefer to bicycle need to own one and find a suitable place to ride it. Soccer, basketball, racquetball, and handball require equipment, an available playing area, opponents, and teammates.

Personal Barriers

Although physical barriers may seem to be major obstacles to exercising, what hampers people more often are *personal* barriers.

"I just don't have the time." The most common obstruction to exercise is a bloated schedule. The process of changing clothes, going to the chosen location, warming up, exercising, cooling down, showering, and dressing can rarely be done in less than thirty minutes if the exercise is meaningful. An hour usually is a more realistic estimate. When commitments to work, home, church, and other assorted duties seem capable of occupying thirty-seven hours per day, carving the better part of an hour out of the pile may require a personal Act of Congress. When the crunch comes—an emergency, a new work assignment, a trip—exercise is usually the first activity to go.

Until personal exercise becomes a positive addiction, schedule it on the calendar—with specific dates and times—on a week-to-week basis. What if you have no time to spare? You may need to do some creative and judicious pruning. The time needed to exercise can be reduced if the activity is done at home. Home exercise videos, a stationary bicycle, or a treadmill are excellent investments, allowing flexibility, privacy, and consistency even when the weather is bad.[7] Placing the bicycle or treadmill near a television or music system can also provide distraction enough to make the time go faster or can allow compulsive types to feel as if they are getting something else accomplished. What if you have no room in the budget for such hardware? Walking or jogging around the block will accomplish the same goals.

Some cooperation among family members may be necessary if only to find creative ways to carve out exercise time. One parent may need to mind the store while the other exercises, and then the next day or night the reverse would occur. Single parents with small children have some of the most challenging scheduling obstacles, but they also are at high risk for chronic fatigue and thus need the energy gain that exercise can provide. Trading child-care duties with another single parent or a cooperative neighbor may be a solution. Some exercise clubs offer child care, if such a club is available and affordable.

Unfortunately, none of these scenarios will happen automatically. Making and taking the time to exercise has to be a deliberate, planned activity. Accepting this and acting accordingly is half the battle.

"Is the gain worth the pain?" For most of us, meaningful exercise feels like hitting ourselves repeatedly with a hammer. It feels so good . . . when we stop. Articles and books about jogging often describe something called "the runner's high"—a blissful experience that overrides the usual negative feelings associated with huffing and puffing. Those who are blessed with the biochemistry that creates a runner's high may skip to the next section. The rest of us need to remember that the good feelings produced by exercise usually occur at other times.

The sensations immediately after the "cool-down" from exercise, especially when it has been vigorous, are usually pleasant—a sense of being invigorated, as if the brain and muscles have been swept of cobwebs. More profound is the change that evolves after *six to eight weeks of consistent exercise.* Improvements in overall energy, productivity, and mood are the rule, but they may not be noticeable immediately. Hang in there, and then compare how you feel after the exercise with how you felt before you began any exercise program. Remember: Even if you don't feel massively energized, you are still making a significant investment in your health.

On a more practical level, you *can* make the exercise experience more enjoyable. No law says you have to choose the most unbearable form of workout. Those who have the opportunity to exercise in one of the more aerobic sports find that the hour (or more) of time spent goes quickly because of the distractions of the game itself.

If you plan to walk or jog, consider what time of day and what environment might be most pleasant. Chugging through the noonday heat or freezing one's posterior before daybreak may invigorate some but discourage the less hardy. One of the best times to exercise outdoors is in the late afternoon or dusk, especially during the summer months. Not only is the temperature more encouraging, but the scenery usually improves with the long shadows. In addition, exercising soon after work can help "blow off steam" and thus reduce the physiological effects of stress.

Traveling by car to a park or a nice neighborhood may also enhance walking, jogging, or cycling. No one wants to worry about being hit by a truck, attacked by an overzealous watchdog, or dragged into the bushes. In addition, the time spent will pass more quickly if you exercise while listening to music or some form of diversion. Small radios or cassette players that can easily be carried or clipped to one's clothing are very affordable.

"I don't know what to do." An important way to minimize pain is to *follow a gradually increasing but regular* pattern of exercise. I routinely advise my patients to pick up one of Dr. Kenneth Cooper's books, like *The Aerobics Program for Total Well-Being* or *The New Aerobics for Women,* for two reasons. First, they provide more detailed background information about the exercise process. More significantly, they provide age-specific charts for each form of aerobic exercise, serving as a blueprint for gradually increased condition-ing over several weeks.

Without this type of information (which is based on measurements of the amount of oxygen consumed during a given activity), one is left without specific goals and guideposts. The lowest levels of exercise should not be overly taxing, and the highest levels should not be attempted before the lower ones are managed comfort-ably. Remember that the intensity of the activity should allow for it to be continued steadily for a prolonged period. If you feel unbearably winded after a few minutes, the activity has probably ceased to be aerobic, and you need to reduce the pace.

People with chronic fatigue syndrome (CFS) must base their exertion on their own tolerance levels. Slow stretching to keep muscles loose is mandatory on a regular basis. Slow walking (even back and forth on the driveway) with frequent rests, if necessary, will still build some stamina, even if at a painfully gradual rate.

"I don't like going out by myself." Some people enjoy using exercise time for personal reflection, when they can clear the mind and think without distractions and mental clutter. For these people, solitude may be a blessing. More often, however, support from and accountability to other people will be a necessary component of a meaningful exercise program.

I happen to enjoy a vigorous game of racquetball as my primary form of exercise. Unfortunately, the only time I can play is at half-past six in the morning. When the alarm goes off at five forty-five, my overwhelming desire is to shut it off and go back to sleep. This impulse is offset by the knowledge that my opponent will think many unpleasant thoughts about me if I don't show up as we arranged the night before. So out I stagger into the dawn's early light, gradually coming to life at some point during the first game.

I have long recognized that I lack the self-discipline to crawl out of bed and jog around the block before the sun comes up. But my desire to avoid losing face is a motivation strong enough to make me do what I would otherwise avoid. This type of "buddy system" can be applied to all forms of exercise. Making a commitment to meet another person at a given time and place on a regular basis can help both people overcome all sorts of personal obstacles.

A particular variation of this social approach to exercise is the aerobic-exercise class. Most private health clubs and some public facilities provide these sessions on a daily basis, usually offering both beginning and more advanced sessions. For the uninitiated, these consist of about an hour spent in a sequence of movements—swinging, swaying, jumping, and jogging to prerecorded music—which typically includes warm-up, full exercise, rhythmic muscle toning, and cool-down. Needless to say, completing the entire sequence is harder than it looks to the casual observer.

Like any form of exercise, aerobic classes have an up side and a down side. A major advantage of group exercise is that one tends to try a bit harder with a live instructor and classmates present than with a prerecorded workout on a television screen. Even though no one is keeping score, the challenge of keeping pace with the instructor can be motivating. The music and the variations of movement can also prevent boredom.

Depending on the circumstances, aerobic classes

also can have disadvantages. A winded, overweight forty-year-old may become discouraged trying to keep up with a sleek, 105-pound instructor who makes it all look so easy. Furthermore, if the class is also populated with "beautiful people" in flashy exercise togs, those who are less well endowed may feel too embarrassed to show up very often. Finally, those whose musical tastes are fairly conservative may feel pummeled by the driving rock-and-roll that aerobic instructors tend to play.

If you plan to engage in group exercise, make sure that the level of exertion required is appropriate for your level of conditioning. More important, don't be afraid to stop and catch your breath if you are having trouble keeping up. Most aerobic-class enthusiasts acknowledge that it takes weeks to be able to fly formation with the instructor for an entire hour.

"I've tried before and I never stay with it." The discouragement of past failures is a big energy drainer for life in general, and it is particularly dangerous here. This mental subterfuge must be dealt with forcefully: "So what?"

For most of us, staying conditioned is an uphill effort all the way, subject to postponement or cancellation at a moment's notice. But so what? If circumstances defeat today's good intentions, mark a new spot on the calendar and try again.

After puffing and straining several times to reach a higher level of conditioning, a week off because of the flu or a crisis at work may cause all of that ground to be lost. It's like starting all over again. But so what? The garden never stays weeded, the garage never remains organized, the car never stays clean. Few things worth doing ever stay done.

"But I've grown out of my exercise gear." So what? Get something that fits and doesn't cost too much. Eventually the smaller clothes will fit again if you stay with it. "But I signed up for the health club six months ago and never went." So what? They really don't care (actually they expect it), and they'll be happy to see you again when you come back. "But my local health club turned out to be an aerobics singles bar." So what? Cancel the membership if you don't like it, or sell it to someone else, and find an exercise companion who doesn't have a hidden agenda.

———————————

Even though the potential excuse list is endless, the benefits of exercise for the tired person are so significant that a deliberate plan of action—and a determination to stay with it for keeps—should be *written down* as soon as possible. This should include:

1. A medical evaluation to check for any possible risks.
2. Acquiring a sensible guide to *gradual* conditioning.
3. Choosing an activity suited for your interest, age, temperament, and the realities of your circumstances.
4. Enlisting the help of family members and friends, if needed, for logistical assistance, companionship, and accountability.
5. Marking exercise times on a calendar and tracking your progress.

6. Refusing to back off when the inevitable circumstances of life arise to make the entire process
more difficult.

The road may be bumpy at times, but it's well
worth the trip.

EIGHT

Nutri-Symptoms

Drainer—Excessive or erratic eating
Gainer—High-quality fuel for your engine

Most people who have been fatigued for a long time eventually wonder whether their dietary habits might be contributing to the problem. Do they have some food allergy that is sapping energy? Do they have a deficiency of a vitamin, mineral, or trace element? Are they tired because they are too heavy or too thin?

Malnutrition

Overt malnutrition (with inadequate protein, calories, or both on a daily basis) is an ongoing problem in the Third World but far less common in well-fed Western cultures. Those particularly at risk of malnutrition in our society are people who are extremely poor (with or without homes), alcoholic, elderly, or mentally ill.

More subtle malnutrition may result from erratic eating patterns in less disturbed or disadvantaged people. Here the problem isn't inadequate fuel, but poor quality or lack of balance. *Excessive alcohol intake,* for example, can result in substitution of the "empty" calories of beer or bourbon for the calories of affordable foods that contain important nutrients. The proverbial "junk-food junkie" can consume hundreds (or thousands) of calories every day in soft drinks, chips, dips, and candy bars and still fail to provide enough protein, vitamins, and minerals to keep the body running smoothly.

Erratic Eating

Fast-paced living leads many to skip breakfast ("not hungry"), grab a snack for lunch ("not much time") and then assemble a colossal meal for dinner—followed by the least active period of the day. *Dieting,* a very common pastime in the Western world, also can be associated with irregular timing and content of meals. In extreme cases, when weight reduction becomes an obsession (anorexia nervosa), the results can be catastrophic.

Nutritional Deficiencies

Specific vitamin and mineral deficiencies that might lead to fatigue are relatively uncommon in our society because our food supply is so abundant and because vitamins are so routinely supplemented in everyday food items. A few cereals claim to contain 100 percent of the recommended daily allowance (RDA) for the most common vitamins and minerals in a single one-ounce serving. Even the manufacturers of Chocolate Covered Godzilla Sugar Bombs will add at least 25 percent of the RDA for some vitamins to every bowl in an attempt to convince the buyer that the product is "part of a nutritious breakfast."

Iron deficiency is probably the most common specific nutrient problem leading to fatigue in our well-fed society. An ongoing supply is necessary for the manufacture of hemoglobin, which carries oxygen molecules within red blood cells. When the iron stored within the body (in the liver, spleen, bone marrow, and other organs) becomes depleted, red cells decrease in size and number, resulting in iron-deficiency anemia. The old ads for Geritol, a proprietary concoction containing iron, used to refer to this as "tired blood"— undoubtedly because the iron-deficient patient does indeed feel weary, even before the red-cell count is affected.

Diagnosing iron deficiency is relatively straightforward. If the deficiency has progressed far enough to cause anemia, a simple blood count will reveal the decreased numbers of red cells and even suggest the cause by demonstrating their small size. Even if anemia has not developed, iron studies are readily available from most laboratories and can be ordered as part of a screening blood panel during the investigation of fatigue.

What is *not* always straightforward is determining the *cause* of the iron deficiency, which may be inadequate supply, excessive demand, or both. Dieters, strict vegetarians, junkaholics, and alcohol abusers all may consume inadequate supplies of the appropriate foods every day. Growing children, adolescents, and menstruating or pregnant women will have increased need for iron.

In men and postmenopausal women, however, iron

deficiency can never be taken at face value. More often than not there has been a steady blood loss, usually from the gastrointestinal (GI) tract. The cause of the bleeding may be trivial or very serious, and thus these people need a thorough evaluation of the food chute from one end to the other. Tests such as a sigmoidoscopy (a look into the final few inches of colon through a flexible scope), a colonoscopy (same thing, but through the entire colon), a barium enema (an x-ray of the colon), and an upper GI series (an x-ray of the esophagus, stomach, and first segment of small intestine) may reveal the source of the leaking red cells.

Vitamin B$_{12}$ deficiency is a relatively rare disorder and, oddly enough, is usually not caused by inadequate amounts of B$_{12}$ in the diet. Since the vitamin is readily available in meat and dairy products (but not in fruits and vegetables), since only minute amounts are needed every day, and since many weeks' worth can be stored in the body, one must work hard at becoming B$_{12}$ deficient through food choices alone. (This will occur, however, on very strict vegetarian diets that do not include eggs or milk.)

More commonly, inadequate levels of B$_{12}$ in the body result from a failure to *absorb* the vitamin, which is the result of a specific disorder of the stomach or the last several inches of small intestine. Since B$_{12}$ is necessary for the production of red cells, a severe anemia may develop over many weeks. This disorder earned the title "pernicious" anemia because of its association with some potentially ruinous problems in the central nervous system, also caused by the lack of B$_{12}$.

Vitamin B$_{12}$ deficiency is usually suspected when a

101

simple blood count demonstrates a low number of very large red cells. Specific tests can confirm the diagnosis, which is easily treated with monthly injections of the vitamin. For some reason, in years past the vitamin B_{12} shot became a lucrative staple in some doctors' offices for "whatever ails ya," a practice now discredited. Nevertheless, occasionally someone enters our office asking for a B_{12} shot because they've been feeling "a little run down."

Some vitamin deficiencies may occur in people with specific diseases or taking certain drugs. Women taking oral contraceptives may become deficient in vitamin B_6, as may those who are taking a prolonged course of the drug isoniazid (INH) to treat tuberculosis. People with certain malabsorption syndromes may be unable to absorb the fat-soluble vitamins (A, D, E, and K). The list of specific interactions between drugs, diseases, and vitamins is lengthy and beyond the scope and purpose of our discussion. Questions about particular situations should be directed to your own physician or better yet to a qualified registered dietitian.[1]

Nutritional Solutions

In chapter 5 we reviewed the subculture that believes fervently that mysterious toxins, dietary deficiencies, and food allergies all play an important role in chronic fatigue. To summarize briefly, I feel that this school of thought lacks credibility in several areas, promotes an obsessive preoccupation with food, and above all seems to presume that the human body is so poorly engineered that it can't function properly without a tacklebox full of food supplements.

In fact, most people who regularly eat reasonable amounts of food from all of the major food groups should not become vitamin deficient. Certain groups of people—infants and growing children, pregnant women, dieters, people recovering from surgery or prolonged illness, and the elderly—may be candidates for supplementation using a basic, all-encompassing multiple vitamin and mineral supplement. In addition, if someone who is chronically tired wants to see if a multivitamin supplement will help, there is little reason to object. (Some patients, running their own individualized "controlled study," have told me that they feel less energetic within a few days off their favorite vitamin.)

Treating iron deficiency is usually straightforward as well. Meats and fish, organ meats such as liver and kidney (if one is so inclined), and whole-grain cereals are excellent dietary sources, although only a small percentage of the iron consumed is actually absorbed. Innumerable vitamin supplements and combinations contain iron, although if a person is truly deficient, a specific iron tablet should be taken two or three times a day initially. Your physician should recommend a particular supplement and monitor the results. (Constipation is common with iron supplements, and some additional fluid and stool softeners may be necessary as well.)

For people who suffer from overt malnutrition, changing circumstances and behavior, not to mention the provision of balanced calories, will lead to a marked improvement in well-being. Unfortunately, this may be more easily said than done. Indeed, the personal, social, and medical conditions associated with malnutrition usually overshadow any specific concern about fatigue.

Energy Drainers, Energy Gainers

Those who feel that the timing and quantity of food affects their energy may need to reconsider their eating patterns. The norm of breakfast at seven o'clock, lunch at noon, and dinner at six o'clock may not work for you. Standard mealtimes simply reflect the most common work and hunger patterns in a given area. They were not handed down on tablets of stone. Some people eat breakfast at six o'clock and then wonder if they are abnormal because they feel weak and hungry by ten o'clock. Other people aren't hungry at all at "normal" mealtimes—and shouldn't feel compelled to eat if that is the case. (However, their presence at a meal, such as a family dinner, may be important for other reasons.) Those who notice sluggishness immediately after a meal and then feel weak and hungry three hours later should consider eating smaller amounts more frequently. A steady but not excessive intake of calories, especially the complex carbohydrates, may not only prevent the ebb and flow of fatigue but actually help reduce excess weight. I mentioned in a previous chapter that much of the excitement about hypoglycemia in years past was not backed by accurate measurements of low blood sugar accompanying fatigue. But the most common dietary solution of frequent small feedings and avoidance of sugar probably helped nonetheless because it promoted smoother delivery of nutrients to the brain (and elsewhere) throughout the day.

In summary, there is no magical, surefire food cure for fatigue. However, remembering a few basic buzzwords will keep most people out of nutritional trouble. The following suggestions parallel the recommendations of the Senate Select Committee on Nutrition and Human Needs, which in 1977 published "Dietary Goals for the United States." These goals are one aspect of an ongoing effort by many governmental and scientific agencies to curb the common "diseases of civilization," such as high blood pressure, heart attack, stroke, and diabetes, which have a dietary link—and which are serious energy drainers.[2]

Sensible Eating

Variety and freshness. The average American supermarket contains a cornucopia of foods that would totally dazzle a visitor from most parts of the world. We have an incredible variety of meats, vegetables, fruits, and grains available at any season. Sampling routinely from all of the groups every day will, for most people, prevent deficiency problems.

In addition, fresh foods are more nutritionally intact than frozen food (though not by much), and both are far more nutritious than canned food. Furthermore, dishes using raw materials prepared with control over some of the less desirable ingredients (such as sugar and salt) are likely to be more wholesome and economical than "Nuke and Serve" concoctions that have already been heavily processed.

Less fat, more complex carbohydrates. We invariably think of some type of meat as the centerpiece of most meals. How many restaurants show meat as a side dish, except at breakfast? Most fast-food joints are built around burgers and fries (or fried chicken). Breakfast has traditionally centered on eggs. And when we order from virtually every menu, the primary decision is the type of meat we want. Unfortunately, as we now know, all of this delicious protein and fat is clogging arteries, expanding waistlines, increasing the risk of diabetes and its major complications, and contributing at least to some forms of cancer.[3]

Complex carbohydrates—such as rice, wheat and other grains, potatoes (before the butter, cheese, and sour cream arrive), pasta, and most fruits and vegetables—have now become the nutritional heroes of the late-twentieth century. They offer more substance with fewer calories and cholesterol, and their undigested remnants (known collectively as fiber) soften the stool and lower the risk of several disorders of the digestive tract. Acknowledging this, the Senate Select Committee recommended that Americans try to consume nearly half of their daily calories from this nutrient category, compared with the more typical 25 percent to 30 percent in previous decades.

Limit the salt and sugar. The dietary sodium found in ordinary table salt and numerous foods is a necessity of life. Fortunately, there is plenty of this element available in all but the most restricted diets. Unfortunately, an overabundance of salt can worsen high blood pressure, make a tired heart's job more difficult, or lead to annoying fluid retention. Fortunately, the vast majority of healthy people can stay out of harm's way by eliminating added salt at the table or at least by tasting the incoming food first to determine whether or not salt is needed. Also, regular intake of salty foods—chips, dips, pickles, cured meats, canned soups, and fast foods—should be limited. Only a small number of people with major heart problems, blood-pressure problems, or kidney problems need more serious restriction.

Similarly, while simple sugars in their various incarnations (such as table sugar, honey, corn syrup, and ingredients in innumerable cereals, soft drinks, and snacks) are not responsible for the decline and fall of Western civilization (as a few writers would suggest), they have little to offer our bodies besides a pleasant experience and a dense flow of calories. The Senate Select Committee recommended a reduction of simple sugars from one-fourth of America's daily calorie input to 10 percent or less. To make this reduction requires some relatively simple adjustments: for example, reducing or eliminating soft drinks from the daily agenda, substituting fruit for desserts (except for sweet and sticky dried fruits), and choosing low-sugar cereals (such as Shredded Wheat or Cheerios) instead of Sugar Bombs.

Sensible Expectations

You're probably beginning to think, *This section sounds like a health-education lecture.* Eat less meat, fat, salt, sugar, sweets, soft drinks, and snacks. Eat a lot of fruits, vegetables, and grains. Go out and buy raw foodstuffs, bake your own bread, don't buy any prepared foods, and spend hours in the kitchen with the "Whole Earth Organic Save the Whales Cookbook." If it tastes good, spit it out, right? Well, not exactly.

The question is this: If you are tired, will this sort of dietary change make you more energetic? The answer is a big maybe. Remember that many people with junky diets have lots of energy. But they'll probably pay for it eventually as they travel down the broad path that leads to the diseases of civilization. Similarly, those who are both tired and married to an erratic, narrow, snack-heavy diet will probably feel better— eventually—as they provide their biochemical engine with better quality fuel.

But how far do you have to go? The nutritional concepts that override all of the others, especially when changes are on the horizon, are *moderation* and *gradual change*. An occasional soft drink, ice cream cone, fast-food meal, or (gasp!) candy bar isn't going to kill anyone. But a steady flow into the stomach is to be discouraged. A small steak won't single-handedly close the coronary arteries. But always ordering the Flaming Buckaroo 16-ounce Porterhouse or the Double Surf and Turf (lobster and filet, dripping with butter) will make a steady contribution to your first heart attack.

Few people are interested in becoming food fanatics who spend a fortune on organic products, sea salt, and fertilized eggs or who can't join their friends for dinner because of paranoia over toxins they may unwittingly consume. But why not try fresh fish for dinner instead of a steak? Why not bake or broil the chicken instead of frying it in a lake of fat? Who decreed that breakfast has to consist of ham and eggs? Why not try the salad bar instead of the double-bacon cheeseburger? Who knows—the experience might be pleasurable. The point is that a gradual, evolutionary change in eating habits is more likely to last than a drastic revision.

A postscript to this section for those who didn't check an earlier footnote: Since this chapter is obviously *not* a comprehensive statement on nutrition, the purchase of a sane book on this subject is highly recommended. A good one is *Jane Brody's Nutrition Book,* which covers a wide gamut of subjects with clarity and common sense. A companion volume, *Jane Brody's Good Food Book* provides a large number of recipes using low-fat, high-carbohydrate ingredients.[4]

TOO MUCH OF A GOOD THING

Having spent the past several pages thinking about nutritional deficiencies as causes of tiredness, the time has come to look at the most common connection between food and fatigue: *overnourishment*. Like it or not, modern technology's efforts to save labor and provide an abundance of calorie-dense food (especially animal-derived foods, which have been a rare commodity for most of the world) have succeeded beyond our wildest dreams. In fact, these two realities of Western civilization virtually guarantee a gradual weight gain throughout adult life unless deliberate steps are taken in the opposite direction. How often these sad refrains have been repeated among friends or at the physician's office: (Fill in the blanks.)

"I haven't changed my eating habits. If anything, I'm eating less. But I'm _____ pounds heavier than I was _____ years ago."

"I've been doing _____ (walking, cycling, Jane Fonda's workout, aerobic sleeping) for the past three months, but nothing has changed."

"I've lost _____ pounds using _____ (Weight Watchers, Jenny Craig, Slim Fast, diet pills, The *National Enquirer*'s Grapefruit and Artichoke

UFO Diet), and within _____ ( ), it all came back."

Like so many other energy drainers, the extent to which the added pounds contribute to chronic fatigue can vary enormously. In seriously overweight people (carrying more than half of their ideal weight as extra fuel), physical complications are inevitable. Blood pressure, cholesterol levels, and blood-sugar levels are all likely to be high, raising the risk for coronary artery disease, heart attacks, heart failure, and their attendant miseries. Bones and joints are more likely to be worn down prematurely or injured in a minor accident. Any surgery can result in major complications. Aside from the various diseases that accompany this much extra padding, the physical labor required to move it from one place to another is exhausting in itself.

The physical drain caused by extra pounds may be less dramatic in the mild to moderately overweight, but the mental and emotional drain is usually significant in all groups. Since the natural tendency for most of us is to gain weight, the point at which the body's appearance and performance leave something to be desired will trigger a psychological trench war.

Eating is easy. Eating feels good. Eating relieves the physical discomfort of hunger. Eating is an occasion to socialize. Eating provides a break in work. Eating can make work less unpleasant. Eating can make recreation more fun. Eating can accompany joy, despair, anger, stress, or contentment.

Conversely, eating less than usual is hard. Eating foods that are not as satisfying is hard. Not eating while others are is hard. Not eating when work is difficult is hard. Eating less or not eating at all when it would feel good will be just about as hard tomorrow as it is today. That thirty-pound weight-loss goal is a long way off. Not eating right now won't provide any immediate satisfaction. And the food is right here, looking and smelling good.

But the clothes aren't fitting well. And what's in the mirror (especially without the clothes) isn't a pretty sight. Come to think of it, my wife's or husband's gaze has been wandering a little in the last few months. And going to the beach is a traumatic event. But summer is a long way off . . .

And so it goes. For so many of us, the weight itself isn't so physically draining, but the endless inner turmoil is a constant energy leak. The desperate search for relief from this conflict has led to a remarkable abundance of weight-reduction mythology, fantasy, and fraud over the decades.

HOW NOT TO LOSE WEIGHT

Diet pills

One of the first patients I saw during my family-practice residency asked the same question every visit: "What are you going to do about my weight?" She was hoping for the arrival of the Holy Grail of weight reduction—a medication that either eliminates interest in food or allows someone to eat whatever looks good while still losing weight. As far as I know, she is still waiting.

The few medications that are used to assist dieters work on the first goal to a mild degree. Their ability to suppress appetite, however, is very limited and does not continue indefinitely. In addition, all have the capacity to elevate pulse rates and blood pressures, and a few are habit forming. The worst of the lot, the amphetamines, are prescribed by a few unscrupulous "diet doctors" who care little about the potential for serious side effects or abuse. The same practitioners are also likely to prescribe high doses of thyroid hormone, which increases the body's metabolic rate (somewhat like changing the idle speed on a car) but with significant risk for toxicity. On the other hand, a new antidepressant, Prozac, appears to decrease appetite without major side effects for most people. Whether this agent will be used widely by dieters remains to be seen.

The problem with diet pills, whether they are mild or dangerous, is that they contribute nothing to behavior or outlook. The ever-present conflict will remain in full force once the medication runs out or becomes ineffective. But these drugs will continue to find a market among those who won't or can't take an active role in the daily decision process.

Operations

Operations such as intestinal bypass, stomach stapling, and the stomach balloon have had a long and colorful history. These procedures have all too often cost more than money. Their effectiveness in creating artificial fullness or preventing food from being absorbed usually is offset by one form of complication or another. More than a few interns and residents have had rich educational experiences managing the metabolic abnormalities of sick bypass patients. In some ways, these procedures are the most drastic measures of all to avoid the long-term struggle between food intake and consequences.

Miracle Foods

Miracle foods or vitamins that "melt pounds away" have basically the same lure as diet pills, but they are even less effective. Check any of the lurid tabloids at the supermarket checkout for further details. A recent entry in our community was the "Fat Magnet" pill, whose creators were unceremoniously busted for fraud. No food can speed metabolism or cause fat cells to shrink. No vitamin prevents the absorption of unwanted calories.

An expensive variation on this theme is the wonderful world of *weight loss injections,* such as HCG (a hormone created by the human placenta during pregnancy) and various other hormonal extracts. Most of these concoctions (sold or shot at a premium) are accompanied by strict eating plans. Guess what actually gets the job done?

Weight-Loss Hardware

Belts, pads, vibrators, or other hardware that claim to compress, jiggle, or otherwise annihilate fat are also ineffective and expensive. The instructions accompanying these pieces of hardware include an eating plan. Need I say more?

Hypnosis

Hypnosis and subliminal-message tapes represent another attempt to avoid the basic conflict. Supposedly, if the subconscious mind can be "programmed" to do the right thing automatically, the rest of the anatomy will follow. Wouldn't it be nice if we didn't have to struggle with decisions so much? Unfortunately, such approaches are notoriously erratic in theory, application, and results. The evidence that subliminal messages (that is, those that can't be consciously heard) actually change behavior is slim indeed, except in the testimonials of those who are selling the products.

Acupuncture

Acupuncture and acupressure are two more passive therapies. For a small fee, some clips in the ear or needles in the right spot or pressure over the right point will curb the appetite. Sound too good to be true? It is. To buy into this form of treatment one must pass into the Twilight Zone of Taoist mysticism, in which the flows of invisible energy are said to affect health and behavior. On the other hand, I suspect that when one has "bought in" to the tune of a few hundred dollars for the treatment, a strong determination to make the investment pay off plays a powerful role—at least for a while.

All of these "solutions" to excessive weight have succeeded far more in separating their desperate customers from their money than from their extra pounds. All of them hinge on a premise that the problem can be solved without decisions, planning, and discipline. All of them are built to a greater or lesser degree on wish fulfillment and denial.

WEIGHT LOSS SECRETS THAT NO ONE LIKES

So what does work? Nothing works. But you or I can work. And if you or I work, then almost anything works. This may sound profoundly dumb, but it follows from some basic principles that lead to long-term success in weight reduction.

Secret #1

There are no magic secrets. Period.

Secret #2

Accept the realities of eating. Whether weight is gained or lost depends on only two variables: how much we take in and how much we use up. First, since the body needs a constant flow of fuel and since it was designed to survive times when fuel isn't available every day, it is very efficient at storing extra fuel for the proverbial rainy day. Unfortunately, the storage capacity is virtually unlimited, but the rate of use is not.

Second, weight will be gained (stored as fat) when more food comes in than is used. Weight will be lost when the body uses more food than is coming in. Despite claims to the contrary, there are some biological limits to the speed with which such gains and losses of fat can take place. Body fluid content, on the other hand, can change rapidly. Most dieters get an initial bonus of a loss of several pounds of fluid when they begin (related to the creation of compounds called ketones, which draw water with them out of the kidneys when fat is first being mobilized). This fluid shift will eventually stabilize as a new steady state is reached, where fluid taken in equals fluid used and eliminated. Otherwise, people who are losing weight would shrivel up like prunes. Once the steady state arrives, the slower, less exciting but true weight loss continues.

Our bodies need to use 3,500 more calories than we eat to lose one pound of fat. Thus, if we work like lumberjacks and eat nothing, we might lose a pound of fat in a day. More realistically, taking in 1000 calories less than used every day will yield a 7000-calorie deficit for a week, resulting in a two-pound loss. Ecstatic claims of thirty-pound weight losses over one month represent some fat and a lot of fluid, as mentioned above. But no one can lose a pound of fat (or anything else) every day for very long by food decisions alone.

Third, the number of calories in various foods has been calculated and is available in numerous books and pamphlets. These figures do not change from year to year or person to person. However, in what is a genuine arena of inequality in the human race, the number of calories used up during the day may vary considerably from person to person or even in the same person during different times of life. It is common for two people to eat the same amount of food and for one to gain from the experience, so to speak, while the other remains unchanged or actually . Furthermore, it requires more calories to maintain muscle than fat, so that the thin, lean person actually can often eat more than the heavy one without gaining weight.

Most people burn their fuel more slowly as they get older. Unfortunately, eating habits rarely change accordingly, resulting in the common phenomenon of middle-age spread. Even more unfortunately, it is very easy to gain weight slowly. Less than twenty calories of excess intake every day—about one teaspoon of sugar's worth—will yield a two-pound weight gain over a year's time, or twenty pounds in a decade.

The body may increase its rate of calorie consumption in some disease states, most notably in the presence of cancer and hyperthyroidism (too much output from the thyroid gland). Attempts to increase the metabolic rate artificially (using supplements or drugs) either don't work or they create a temporary disease state of their own. Don't even try them.

Fourth, it is very difficult to lose weight by exercising alone, without a change in eating patterns. A 200-pound person walking four miles per hour (a reasonably brisk rate) will burn fewer than 250 calories in a half hour—enough to mobilize fewer than two ounces of fat, all things being equal. We mention this *not* to discourage exercise, but to *prevent* discouragement when several weeks of exercising daily without altering food intake doesn't change the weight that much. Also note that increasing exercise will build muscle mass, which is more dense (and thus weighs more) than fat. It is thus possible for someone who increases exercise quite a bit to become thinner in appearance without seeing much weight loss.

Secret #3

Accept the fact that you can't eat all the food you would like to eat. If this is indeed the case, then the idea of eating what we need instead of what is available or what we would like should not be quite such an unpleasant one. This observation also applies to the

117

mythology of the Clean-Plate Club. Some of us can't stand the thought of food "going to waste," so we feel compelled to eat something destined for the garbage disposal, even though we are perfectly full. But remember: Food that goes down the sink doesn't add to a weight problem, which is the more serious form of "going to waist."

Secret #4

Small amounts of food inform the brain that hunger is satisfied just as fast as large amounts of food. Furthermore, eating quickly doesn't relieve hunger any faster than eating slowly. Therefore, eating a small amount of food slowly can be just as satisfying as eating a large amount quickly. Not only is food enjoyed and indigestion avoided, but fewer calories are taken in.

Secret #5

Don't think of "going on a diet." This phrase has all the appeal of the words "going on a budget," which in turn is like saying "going to jail." "Going on a diet" implies that a sentence is to be served for past misdeeds, and when the punishment is over, life can go on as before. Wrong. If life going on as usual led to twenty or eighty extra pounds, then the same behavior started over will yield the same results.

Accept the fact that managing food (like managing money) is a lifelong process and that it will probably be a lifelong difficulty. Coming to terms with this reality, and acting accordingly, can be liberating. Instead of wasting time and energy on all of the schemes and pills and weird therapies that are merely forms of denying the problem, useful effort can be exerted toward the goal of a leaner, meaner, more efficient body.

Secret #6

Pick a food-management plan and stick to it. Examine several food-management plans (no one said the *D* word), select one you can live with, and persist with it like a pit bull. Please note that *any* food plan will result in weight reduction if fewer calories are taken in than used. Even bizarre, stupid, irrational food plans work if they lead to fewer calories in than out. Since the bookstores are filled with bizarre, stupid, irrational food plans, be careful what you pick. Since the yellow pages contain ads for many practitioners who charge a lot of money for bizarre, stupid, irrational food plans, choose carefully the person to whom you say, "Tell me what to do and I'll do it." But if you have made a reasonable choice, stay with it for keeps.

Among the various possibilities for food-management plans, the one called "I'll just try to eat less" works for a few people. Very few. The rest are advised to choose something more formal, more concrete, more specific. Some options include the following:

Books. Examples include *Jane Brody's Nutrition Book,* already mentioned in this chapter. It contains an excellent, sensible section on weight reduction. *The New American Diet* by Sonja and William Connor focuses more on specific recipes, but is sane and sensible.[5] *Fit or Fat* by Covert Bailey is more motivational than food-specific but is a useful resource.[6]

Books have the advantage of minimal expense. (They can be borrowed from the library if money is an issue, although it is nice to own a copy of one's chosen resource.) They also allow for more privacy during the weight-reduction process. But that advantage can also be a detriment if motivation can't be sustained from within. Much can be gained (and much weight lost) when there is *accountability* as well. Like it or not, many of us will do things just to save face. (Remember the same thing was said about exercise.) Furthermore, we can find much encouragement in seeing the progress of others or hearing about their struggles or learning about something that worked for another person. All of the following resources take advantage of the accountability factor.

National organizations. National groups with hundreds of local chapters include *Weight Watchers* and *TOPS* (Take Off Pounds Sensibly). Both of these organizations disseminate materials and methods that health professionals recognize as sane and sensible. They are also far less expensive than some of the more aggressive programs (see below). For these to work, however, one must be reasonably comfortable with the local group and its members.

In addition, local chapters of *Overeaters Anonymous* help deal with the drives and emotions that can play a major role in weight gain.

Individual consultation. Consultation with a registered dietitian is a viable alternative for the person who doesn't care for the group approach. In addition, the individual attention allows for a more streamlined approach as specific problems are attacked. (This is the nutritional equivalent of the private ski lesson.) More can be accomplished in a given session when the instructor is paying attention to one person instead of a group.

A local hospital may provide this service, or a dietitian may work in conjunction with a private physician or medical group. Some work on their own in the community. As we mentioned previously, beware of "nutritionists" who offer big promises, unusual food plans, and food supplements.

Franchise programs. Programs like Nutri-Systems and Jenny Craig offer a more comprehensive approach. After paying an initial fee based on the anticipated weight loss, the enrollee buys food from the program for several weeks while attending classes and small groups. Follow-up continues after the transition back to store-bought food, and typically there is a partial refund if the weight loss is maintained for a designated period of time.

These types of programs work very well for the person who doesn't want to be hassled—at least in the beginning—with a lot of decisions about types and amounts of food. (Most of us are not enthralled with the idea of weighing out portions of food or playing with measuring cups and calculators at every meal.) The "no-brain" approach of eating prescribed amounts of food provides a general idea of what constitutes a 1000- or 1500-calorie intake. Obviously, at some point one must learn the economics of food, but this can be done over time during the classes.

One major disadvantage of a franchise program is

its cost. Several hundred dollars will be spent (mostly on the food, which is obviously going to cost more than store-bought food). On the other hand, if the process is successful on a long-term basis, the money spent will be well worth it. Another aspect to consider is the palatability of the food. Is the cuisine going to become a stumbling block after the novelty wears off? The most important pitfall of this approach is the failure to follow through when it's time to "do it yourself." Remember one of the previous secrets—this is a lifetime process, and the job isn't over once the desired weight is attained.

The commando program. A protein-sparing fast is available in some communities. Here, no food is eaten for several weeks. In order to prevent muscle wasting, a few hundred calories of protein must be taken every day in a more or less tolerable drink. *This approach is potentially dangerous and must be carried out only under medical supervision.* An initial physical examination is necessary and ongoing monitoring of certain blood tests while the fast is in progress. After the supervised "refeeding" period, most programs continue prolonged follow-up.

Assuming that there are no medical risks, this go-for-broke approach is best for someone with a large amount of weight to lose, especially if other programs have been unsuccessful and if there is a medical problem (such as high blood pressure or cholesterol) that will benefit from a major change in body size. Although these programs are expensive, the cost is sometimes partially covered by insurance if the treatment is recommended by a physician. The daily ration of protein drink can become almost unbearably monotonous, but for some people the dramatic weight loss more than compensates.

The greatest pitfall of a protein-sparing fast is its aftermath. If ongoing, long-term follow-up does not continue for several months (or longer), all of the gains may be lost (or the losses gained, depending on how you look at it).

In addition to nutritional input, counseling therapy may be needed. In fact, for some people, counseling may be more important than information about food. As I noted earlier, we often eat for nearly every reason other than hunger. All sorts of issues may be feeding the problem, so to speak, and the most clever weight-reduction program will not accomplish anything until these issues are addressed. Anxiety and depression, both very common in our society, are often accompanied by disorders in eating patterns.

When eating is an obsession or when it leads to extraordinarily high weights (over 350 pounds) or when it occurs in extremes of binges and fasts (especially if measures such as vomiting or laxative use have been taken), counseling is mandatory. Indeed, multidisciplinary eating-disorder programs and even hospitalization may be necessary when an extreme preoccupation with weight leads to the dangerous disorder known as anorexia nervosa.[7]

NINE

Side Effects

Drainer—*Prescription, nonprescription, and "recreational" drugs*
Gainer—*A change, when needed*

One of the most important reasons for chronic fatigue—
one that should never be overlooked—is an adverse
effect from medication. Fatigue can result from prescription as well as nonprescription drugs, and from
"recreational" drugs such as tobacco and alcohol.

ENERGY-DRAINING PRESCRIPTION AND NONPRESCRIPTION DRUGS

How much fatigue a drug will cause will depend
not only on its own characteristics but also on the person
taking it and the *length* of its use. Obviously, a drug
taken only for a few days is hardly likely to cause
chronic fatigue. And certain types of long-term medications may cause fatigue only for a short time. Others may
not cause fatigue until they have been used for a while.

Determining which drug might be causing the
fatigue is a difficult process, especially in elderly
patients who may be taking six or seven prescription

drugs. Unfortunately, figuring out whether fatigue is actually caused by one or more medications is harder than it might sound. At times it is necessary to discontinue a drug for a while, see whether the symptom improves, and then start it again. Obviously, this should be done only with the approval of the doctor who first prescribed it, because abrupt discontinuation can be hazardous in some situations. If a clear relationship can be demonstrated—tired on the drug, better when off it—your doctor should try to find an alternative medication.

The following list of energy-draining drugs includes those that tend to be used continuously or repeatedly for weeks or months at a time.

Antihistamines

Antihistamines, common remedies for colds and allergies, can cause immediate drowsiness or prolonged fatigue. They may be sold as single agents, such as diphenhydramine (Benadryl) or chlorpheniramine (Chlor-Trimeton), or in combination with decongestants (Actifed, Contac, Drixoral, Comtrex, Dimetapp, etc.), which by themselves *rarely* produce this effect.[1] While these agents generally are effective in relieving the symptoms of colds and allergies, they do not directly affect any virus.

Interestingly, there is no way to predict who will react adversely to what. Some adverse effects can be avoided if the medication is tailored to the problem. For routine colds, a simple decongestant, such as pseudoephedrine (Sudafed), will usually provide satisfactory relief without any drowsiness at all. For nasal allergy (where the sneezing and runny nose is not caused by a virus but is a reaction to pollen, molds, dust, or some other airborne troublemaker), antihistamines are far more effective. To prevent drowsiness and fatigue, very often the antihistamine can be taken in the evening or at bedtime, with a decongestant alone doing its best during the day.

Better yet, certain antihistamines, like clemastine (Tavist), terfenadine (Seldane), and especially astemizole (Hismanal), rarely produce any side effects at all. Unfortunately, for reasons related entirely to economics and not to product safety, these agents are available only by prescription and are much more expensive.

Drugs That Lower Blood Pressure

Hypertension—high blood pressure, not a state of being "hyper" or tense—is both common and potentially dangerous. Very often medications are deemed necessary to coax blood pressure into a desirable range. Several categories of drugs are available, and some are more likely to cause fatigue than others.

Many of the *beta blockers*, which slow the heart rate and decrease the forcefulness of each contraction, are well-known fatigue makers. Propranolol (Inderal) and nadolol (Corgard) are known for this effect, while atenolol (Tenormin) and acebutolol (Sectral) are far less likely to produce it. Others in the group are more difficult to predict. Clonidine (Catapres), which affects the nervous system's control of blood pressure, is very often sedating. Reserpine is so famous for causing fatigue and depression that it is rarely prescribed any more. Methyldopa (Aldomet) is another sedating drug that is not used much today, although those who have done well with it for years do not need to change to something else.

Blood-pressure medications that do *not* usually cause fatigue are the *diuretics* ("water pills"), which decrease the body's fluid volume; the so-called *ACE inhibitors*, like captopril (Capoten), enalapril (Vasotec), and lisinopril (Prinivil and Zestril), which inhibit the production of a blood-pressure-raising hormone in the kidneys; and the relatively new group called *calcium channel blockers*, such as verapamil (Calan or Isoptin), nifedipine (Procardia), and diltiazem (Cardizem). Because of more favorable side effects profiles and once-daily dosing schedules, many of the ACE inhibitors and calcium channel blockers are started more frequently than the older, more sedating drugs.[2]

One important reminder: In some people, especially elderly people who have had high blood pressure for a long time, lowering the blood pressure alone will produce fatigue, at least for a while. Therefore, it is not a good idea to give up on a medication until enough time has passed to judge its effects and side effects.

Antidepressants

Ironically, antidepressants are often the very agents prescribed to treat chronic fatigue caused by depression. The right agent in the right patient can produce a dramatic improvement, but because many of these drugs are sedating, they can also worsen fatigue, particularly at first. As with blood pressure medications, it is wise not to bail out too quickly because the side effects are often transient.

Tranquilizers

Since drugs that reduce anxiety, such as alprazolam (Xanax), diazepam (Valium), and lorazepam (Ativan), are by definition sedating, they are ideal candidates to produce fatigue. In some people they produce fatigue by relieving the nervousness that accompanies an underlying depression, allowing the depression to express itself more fully. In other people, severe anxiety by itself is fatiguing, so both are improved by these drugs—for a while. The well-publicized risk with all tranquilizers is their ability to produce dependence, both psychological and physical, when used for long periods of time. The proper and improper use of tranquilizers is discussed further in chapter 12. If you are taking one of these drugs on a regular basis and are feeling tired, discuss the fatigue with your doctor.

It should be noted that a relatively new drug used to treat anxiety, buspirone (Buspar), appears to be both minimally sedating and not habit forming. However, since it relieves symptoms rather gradually, the extent to which it will be used in the coming decade remains to be seen.

Drugs for Neurological Disorders

Drugs used to treat epilepsy and Parkinson's disease can produce fatigue. Often difficult choices must be made between the benefits and drawbacks of medications when these types of problems are under treatment. Obviously, control of seizures is a high priority for anyone, but most anticonvulsants, like phenytoin (Dilantin) and carbamazepine (Tegretol), can produce sluggishness and drowsiness, especially when blood levels are high. Keeping track of blood levels and adjusting dosing schedules can alleviate this problem. *Under no circumstances should any treatment for epilepsy be changed without consulting the physician involved.* The most common cause of an unexpected seizure is reducing or stopping medication.

Similarly, the trade-off between the physical limitations of Parkinson's disease (especially tremor and rigid movements) and the side effects of the drugs that control them can be a major issue. One articulate patient of mine became distressed by the progression of coordination problems arising from her Parkinson's disease. After consultation with a neurologist, her medications were "beefed up" in an effort to turn the tide. Unfortunately, the cure proved to be worse than the disease, with significant nausea and fatigue. Eventually we had to return to square one—still seeing gradual deterioration, but at least she was able to eat and stay awake.

Pain Relievers

Pain relievers that are *narcotics* (or related to narcotics) are inherently sedating. When these pain relievers are taken over a long period of time, this effect is less noticeable because the body becomes accustomed to the drug and its effects are less impressive. Anyone who takes narcotic pain relievers, especially codeine and its derivatives hydrocodone (Vicodin, Zydone, Bancaps) and oxycodone (Percodan, Percocet, Tylox), for a prolonged period probably has a lot of reasons for fatigue.

Chronic pain syndromes are draining and

frequently are associated with depression. Narcotics in these situations are a surefire dead end, creating not only negative side effects but also a negative relationship with at least one physician. Getting off these drugs and working on the pain usually is a multidisciplinary task, which may require help from a primary-care physician, a physical therapist, a psychiatrist, or a psychologist. Frequently a team approach, like those in pain clinics often associated with university hospitals, is most appropriate.

Drugs for Intestinal Disorders

Drugs used to treat certain intestinal disorders can cause fatigue. Medications for nausea, such as prochlorperazine (Compazine) and promethazine (Phenergan), are inherently sedating, but fortunately people rarely need them for very long. The antinausea patch Transderm Scōp is a popular treatment for seasickness but is extremely sedating for some people. Metoclopramide (Reglan), which is used to relieve recurrent heartburn, is often taken for months at a time, often resulting in fatigue.

Checking the Medicine Chest

Similarly, common *antispasmodics* used to treat the cramps of irritable bowel can be sedating, especially for people who use them over a long period of time. Some antispasmodics, including Donnatal and Librax, actually contain small doses of tranquilizers. Even the pure cramp relievers like hyosciamine (Levsin) and dicyclomine (Bentyl) can cause fatigue.

If you think one of your medications may be causing fatigue, talk about it with your doctor. Never make changes without medical supervision; stopping some medications could cause serious damage to your system. With your doctor's supervision, you may discover a chain reaction leading to fatigue, even if one single medication isn't itself the primary cause. For example, the chronic use of an anti-inflammatory drug to treat arthritis might cause ongoing blood loss into the intestine, which in turn eventually produces a tiring iron-deficiency anemia. In some patients (especially the elderly), a simple diuretic to treat high blood pressure can lead to an impressive collection of biochemical abnormalities that may express themselves in fatigue.

If you and your doctor suspect that a certain drug is causing fatigue, change only that drug until you both are sure it either is or is not causing the fatigue. Then proceed to change another one. Don't make more than one change at a time.

Finally, be careful not to over-interpret symptoms. Some people assume too quickly that one or more discomforts are being produced by a medication (especially if they're not excited about taking it in the first place). They may lose a potential benefit if they discontinue their medication too quickly.

ENERGY-DRAINING "RECREATIONAL" DRUGS

Responding to energy-draining medications may be a challenge, but dealing with "recreational" drugs is like entering a war zone. Not only can some of these ever-popular chemical agents suck the life out of their users, but they don't relinquish their prey easily.

Energy Drainers, Energy Gainers

Tobacco

Smoking is not only the most common form of drug habit in the world, but it also is one of the most difficult to break. The Tobacco Institute and the various corporate giants that support it have deemed smoking to be an "adult social custom." They have also battled ferociously to convince anyone who will listen that smoking is not even a habit, let alone an addiction. While their rhetoric suggests that smoking is one of life's simple pleasures that can be started and stopped at will, even a casual poll of the next ten smokers you meet (or yourself, if you smoke) will flatly prove otherwise.

About once a year I talk to a patient who claims to smoke once in a while at a party and otherwise can take it or leave it. All of the other smokers I meet light up compulsively several times a day, often without conscious awareness of their behavior. If I recite a list of the wonderful effects of tobacco smoke, I may influence the frontal lobes, where rational thinking takes place. But the chemicals in cigarette smoke (especially nicotine) have me beat because they are entrenched in the more primitive areas of the brain.

One reason for this is that nicotine has the unusual property of being stimulating and relaxing at the same time. Another is that the lungs "mainline" nicotine directly into the bloodstream, producing a powerfully reinforcing "hit" on the central nervous system with every puff. A third reason is that the smoking behavior is cued by dozens of everyday events: picking up the phone, getting into the car, having a cup of coffee, to name a few. You don't have to hide from the police or anyone else to smoke, although fewer public places now tolerate tobacco pollution.

The most pathetic patients in any medical practice are the cigarette addicts who must struggle to quit when circumstances like a heart attack or worsening chronic lung disease or a pregnancy force the issue. Yet, stopping is a Herculean task.

It is here that chronic fatigue enters the picture in one of two ways. The most obvious energy drainers related to tobacco are the numerous diseases it causes or aggravates, especially chronic bronchitis and emphysema, which can force the longtime smoker to struggle for every breath. But equally draining is the internal warfare caused by feeling the obvious effects of the smoke but wanting more anyway—a true hallmark of addiction. Each puff generates a mental indictment of one's ability to think straight. The smoker's life is aggravated by the hacking and wheezing and phlegm that invariably accompany this adult social custom.

Kicking the Habit

Dealing with tobacco addiction requires some of the same decisions needed to lose weight. The necessary ingredients include a plan, accountability, and some reinforcement.

Method. The specific method of quitting may vary from a simple decision to stop on a certain date (New Year's Day, birthday, or any other occasion will do) to a formal program. Local hospitals, national organizations, such as the American Lung Association, and for-profit organizations, such as Smokenders, run local seminars on an ongoing basis. A program has the advantage of being more specific and definite, especially when compared to a vague statement such as, "I need to start cutting down." By the way, whether the cigarettes are gradually phased out over time or dropped cold turkey doesn't matter as much as whether or not there is a specific quitting date on the calendar.

Passive therapies, such as acupuncture or hypnosis, are far less reliable over the long haul than approaches that involve the conscious mind. These methods tend to succeed because some hard-earned cash has been spent on them, reinforcing an internal commitment that "This had better work . . ."

Accountability. Accountability is a way of borrowing some willpower. The decision to quit needs to be broadcast far and wide, among family, friends, and co-workers so that in a moment of weakness the urge to smoke will be countered by an equally powerful desire not to look like a spineless fool. Those who smoke need to be asked to light up somewhere else, and by all means they must refrain from offering cigarettes to the person who is quitting.

Reinforcement. Reinforcement for the quitting process can and should come from a number of directions. The first and most important is an inner conviction, backed by some emotion, that this is the right decision. All too often smokers facing their day of reckoning do so with considerable grieving—"Do I really have to give up my seven-minute vacations?" When my patients are struggling with this, I lay down the challenge to identify themselves as nonsmokers, not as smokers who are refraining through some exercise of willpower. I also ask them to think about their ongoing financial support of the tobacco industry, which grows wealthy at their expense and could not care less about their health. Furthermore, if the idea of squandering their God-created body fails to ignite adequate concern, I have no qualms about raising the specter of loved ones left behind by the smoker's premature trip to Forest Lawn. If smoking behavior is driven by emotions that over-power reason, then emotions will usually be necessary for a counterattack.

Other forms of reinforcement can best be summa-rized by the biblical advice regarding temptation: Flee it rather than fight it. It is much easier to avoid doing the wrong thing if the wrong thing isn't readily available. For openers, the living arrangements should be smoke free. Ashtrays, lighters, and any other tobacco parapher-nalia need to be trashed. Anyone in the dwelling who continues to smoke should be asked politely to do so on the back porch.

The workplace also should be cleared of smoke, if necessary. Fortunately, many if not most employers (particularly large corporations) have created designated smoking areas and left the remainder of the office or factory off limits. Agencies that regulate work environ-ments generally accept the dictum that *no one should have to inhale someone else's smoke while on the job*, and they will tend to back anyone who forces the issue.

Recreational activities may be more difficult to manage. Restaurants, fortunately, have designated non-smoking areas. Sporting events, bars, and bowling alleys, on the other hand, usually are tobacco infested, and some discretion may be needed during the vulnerable early days of smoke-free life. Harder still are those social events where the smoking friends gather, unless you're the host, in which case a nice "Thank you for not smoking" sign may embellish your entryway. Choosing dinners and parties carefully and even making some new, nonsmoking friends may be necessary for success.

Alcohol

Alcohol can also be an important energy drainer, for any number of reasons. Even though many people find that alcohol in modest amounts adds a pleasant dimension to a meal or a social event, the potential for disaster looms in the distance, even for the occasional user. The first issue to consider is this: How much is reasonable and how much is "one too many"? Some of my patients define "moderate" alcohol use as a six-pack every night after work. Other "moderate" drinkers shun any booze on weeknights but then spend every Saturday and Sunday inebriated.

Medical professionals generally agree that a maximum of two drinks in twenty-four hours should not be expected to cause physical complications. (A "drink" here is defined as a twelve-ounce can of beer, a four-ounce glass of wine, or one ounce of distilled spirits in any form. This concept does *not* apply to the pregnant woman, someone with liver disease, or any of several other conditions that might be adversely affected by alcohol. If in doubt, check with your doctor.) On the other hand, even the occasional alcohol user who stays within the two-drink limit will experience temporary sedation, a lapse in intellectual function, and possibly a night of disrupted sleep as a consequence of imbibing.

This may prove to be inconsequential. But it may also lead to a missed opportunity, a slip of the tongue, or an accident, any of whose long-term effects could be life changing.

The regular alcohol user will eventually have plenty of reasons to feel tired, generally in proportion to the amount of alcohol consumed every day. The empty calories in all those drinks have to go somewhere, and excess weight may result. On the other hand, if the liquid calories displace real food too often, some forms of malnutrition will eventually develop. Blood pressure tends to become erratic, and a physician unaware of the alcohol situation may prescribe medication to control it; as we have seen, many antihypertensive medications cause long-term fatigue.

The more severe medical problems caused by chronic alcohol abuse are horrendous. The heart muscle may become damaged (alcoholic cardiomyopathy), leading to overt failure. The pancreas may become inflamed (pancreatitis), a highly painful and often recurrent condition. Persistent irritation of the liver can lead to scarring (cirrhosis) or outright liver failure. Complications include the accumulation of gallons of fluid in the abdomen (called ascites), dilated esophageal veins that can rupture and cause sensational bleeding episodes, major disruption of the brain, and more. When these occur, fatigue is the least of one's problems.

The fatigue problems created by chronic alcohol use, however, extend well beyond the medical realm. Arguments and physical violence are alcohol's regular traveling companions, as are impairments in work or outright loss of one or more jobs. The flashing red lights in the rearview mirror of the inebriated driver are just the beginning of some tiring legal problems—but these are preferable to a long hospital stay or a trip to the morgue. A witty but also poignant description of an alcoholic's life in the book of Proverbs begins,

> Who has woe? Who has sorrow?
> Who has strife? Who has complaints?
> Who has needless bruises? Who has bloodshot
>   eyes?
> Those who linger over wine . . .
>
> (Prov. 23:29–30)

The factors that lead to alcohol abuse have been the subject of considerable research and discussion and will not be reviewed here. Unlike smoking, in which addictive behavior is virtually universal, alcohol use for many is casual and occasional. For some, however, a genetic predisposition contributes to compulsive drinking, even in the face of terrible consequences. All too often, even while seeing that time, money, health, and energy are being lost because of alcohol consumption, the most common response is denial: "I really don't have a problem."

So when should alcohol be considered a problem rather than a pleasant diversion? Long before jobs are lost, families break up, and liver functions change. The time to become concerned is when having a drink is no longer a take-it-or-leave-it proposition, when one feels that "something is missing" if alcohol isn't available in a given situation, or when alcohol contributes in any way to a disturbance in one's life. When one of these occurs, the response must be total abstention, not merely cutting back. Once drinking is an issue, trying to become a "moderate" or "social" drinker is like trying to be "just a little bit pregnant." Needless to say, no reputable program for treatment of alcoholism strives toward "moderate" drinking.

When it is time to quit and when abstaining is a struggle to any degree, the services of a counselor, program, or support group *on a long-term basis* are a necessity, because the inclination to drink, and drink in excess, *does not go away*. Alcohol-recovery groups sponsored by churches, Alcoholics Anonymous groups, and more elaborate substance-abuse programs all stress the need for permanent accountability and acknowledgment that no one can solve the problems alone. Dependence on God and support from others who have fought the same battle are necessary ingredients for lasting success.

Other Energy-Draining Drugs

Often alcohol abuse is but one component of a more broad-based problem. Overuse of prescription drugs, as noted earlier, is a surefire energy drainer. But once one begins looking for better living through illegal chemistry, the route to fatigue and outright catastrophe is short indeed. Ongoing marijuana use impairs intellectual function and damages the lungs more efficiently than cigarettes. Hallucinogenic drugs and PCP can create a temporary psychosis (which in a few pathetic cases becomes permanent). The all-consuming drive to obtain the next dose of cocaine or heroin, not to mention the physiologic roller coaster these drugs create, rapidly depletes energy—but usually the more dramatic problems need immediate attention.

Energy Drainers, Energy Gainers

Needless to say, becoming clean and sober after using street drugs for any length of time is a full-blown project, requiring the services of a well-organized, ongoing program. The most important step is facing the fact that drugs are in the driver's seat, and that the vehicle they're driving is heading for a cliff. Then, picking up the phone and calling for help can prevent a disaster.

TEN

Mr. Sandman, Bring Me Some Sleep

Drainer—No rest for the weary
Gainer—Normalized sleep

Many cases of chronic fatigue are accompanied by sleep disorders of variable severity, but how they are related is not always clear. For example, it may be difficult to tell whether lack of productive sleep is the cause of the fatigue or is a component of another problem altogether. This chapter will focus on sleep that is inadequate in hours, quality, or both.

ACUTE SLEEP DISTURBANCES

Acute disturbances in sleep are usually the by-product of some unpleasant but short-term event. An all-nighter during final exams, a new baby, an acute illness, an oversized meal, intercontinental travel, a strange bed, a child's first date—all of these disrupt sleep. A few of these episodes may be an appropriate occasion for a short-acting sleeping medication (see below), but more often they signal a need to deal with a problem during waking hours. Of these examples, all but one— the new baby—usually affect only one or two nights of sleep. Let's take a closer look at sleep disturbances caused by having a new baby. If you don't have small children at home, skip the next few paragraphs.

Parents of newborns are virtually guaranteed sleep interruptions as their offspring awaken every few hours to be fed. An illness, colic, or any other source of discomfort can extend nocturnal crying into what seems like hours on end. In addition, some infants have a tendency to reverse their day-night cycle: they can sleep through anything when the sun is up, then they fuss and sputter relentlessly when it's time for their parents to sleep. During the first few months, there are only a few ways to maximize the precious hours of sleep at night.

One maneuver that may help is allowing the baby to sleep in a nearby room. New parents often feel more secure if their bundle is in a bassinet within arm's length. Unfortunately, all babies rustle around during the night, uttering numerous grunts and other "false alarms" that awaken parents even when a feeding isn't needed. Except in highly unusual circumstances, even the youngest newborn will sound off loudly when it's feeding time. I always tell parents to make whatever sleeping arrangements they prefer but to relax about putting the infant in the next room if no one is getting any sleep. I also recommend that little ones be brought into bed with Mom and Dad only on rare occasions, if at all. Children grow strongly attached to this arrangement, and I have watched parents go through considerable teeth gnashing as they try to break an older child of the habit of crawling into bed with them at all hours of the night.

A second tip is to keep the feeding times short and

sweet during the night. Some infants love to nurse for hours on end, but virtually all of mother's milk has been dispensed after ten minutes on each side. The rest is socializing, so to speak, which is better done during daylight hours. Occasionally a baby will continue to cry during the night, despite feeding, changing, rocking, singing, pacing the floor, and another feeding. During those character-building moments, it is quite all right to set the little bundle back into the crib for fifteen minutes, walk away for a while to relax (if possible), and then try again. If the child hasn't gone to sleep, usually he or she will have expended enough energy to become drowsy with a little more rocking. And if that doesn't work, try a short drive in the car; there is something about the gentle jostling of the back seat that works when all else fails.

Finally, when is it time to work on putting an end to the feeding at two o'clock in the morning? For the first three months, newborns need the night feedings, but once they reach nine months, they should be snoring through the night without interruption. If they continue to demand food in the middle of the night, parents should plan for a "commando weekend." Pick two consecutive nights when sleep is not a premium, and make sure the infant is not fighting an illness of some sort. Tuck the baby in, say goodnight, close the door, and don't go back unless absolutely necessary. What may seem like endless hours of wailing must be ignored (a couple of good midnight movies may be necessary). Relenting even after three or four hours (a rare demonstration of infant stamina) is disastrous, because the baby learns, to quote Sir Winston Churchill, "Nevah give up!" The parents who hang tough will be rewarded with uninterrupted sleep after one or at most two nights.

CHRONIC SLEEP DISORDERS

Chronic problems with sleep (that is, lasting more than three weeks and not caused by young children) can have both physical and psychological origins. Physical hindrances may arise from the circumstances surrounding sleep, particularly when they change from a well-established pattern. A bedroom can be too hot or cold, light or dark, noisy or quiet. Some people need dead silence to fall asleep, while others feel more comfortable with some soft noise droning in the background. Some sleep best on a firm mattress, while others prefer a water bed. Determining one's ideal conditions may require some trial and error, especially when the needs of another in the room or in the bed must be considered.

Other physical problems that can banish the sandman include various *diseases* and the *effects of medications*. Chronic heart or lung disease may keep a person awake with shortness of breath. Intestinal disorders may generate some unpleasant cramps or burning during the night. Chronic pain from any number of sources may inhibit sleep. Drugs and medications, including caffeine, alcohol, nicotine, diet pills, and decongestants, can produce insomnia. Withdrawal from narcotics, sedatives, and (ironically) some sleeping pills not only can keep people awake but also can tempt them to use the problem drug again in order to get some sleep.

One particular disorder that is gathering more attention is sleep apnea. (The word *apnea* literally means "without breath.") Certain anatomy problems,

144

including obesity and large tonsils, lead to irregularities in breathing—dangerously long pauses between breaths. Heavy snoring and profound sleepiness during the day are irritating components of the syndrome. Potentially more worrisome are falls in blood-oxygen levels during the pauses between breaths, sometimes resulting in heart-rhythm changes. Evaluation and treatment of suspected sleep apnea should be done by a consultant well versed in sleep disorders, usually a lung specialist (pulmonologist) with additional training in this area.

Certain *behaviors* can lead to sleep problems. The "night owl" may actually have a disorder called the delayed-sleep-phase syndrome. He or she may be unable to fall asleep until the late-late-late show is over (between three o'clock and six o'clock in the morning), but then sleeping as long as necessary is no problem— unless one has one of those minor inconveniences known as a job. This problem can be treated during a week off work by delaying bedtime two or three hours each day until a more normal bedtime is reached.

Variable work shifts can turn sleeping patterns inside out. If the job calls for these to rotate periodically, it is easier to change in a clockwise direction (for example, from evening to night shift) than the other way around. *Air travel* back and forth across several time zones disrupts sleeping patterns. Adjustment time may require as many days as the number of time zones crossed, with adjustment from west-to-east travel taking longer than the other direction.[1]

An important cause of disturbed sleep is *depression,* which will be reviewed in detail in the next chapter. The mechanisms that keep depressed people awake much of the night or cause them to stay in bed all day are not merely their sad moods or agitation over life. Biochemical mechanisms are usually at work too, as demonstrated by the improvement in sleep seen in many who are treated with antidepressant medications (drugs that, incidentally, do not work as sleeping aids in the general population).

HOW TO GET ENERGY-GAINING SLEEP

Given the fact that there may be many reasons why sleep is disturbed and disrupted, what approaches are appropriate to bring some order back into the hours spent in bed? The first solution should *not* be to call your doctor for a few sleeping pills, except perhaps for a very specific and short-term sleep-robber such as a family crisis. Over-the-counter agents are basically antihistamines whose drowsy side effects are being put to work. Prescription sleeping agents in the benzodiazepine family (the most common being Dalmane, Restoril, and Halcion) all work well and are the agents of choice if one is going to use anything at all. Dalmane remains in the bloodstream longer than the others and is the most likely of the three to cause sedation the next day. Halcion, on the other hand, is very short acting and essentially gone by morning. However, doses over .25 milligrams every night on a long-term basis have been associated with significant emotional problems. Indeed, prolonged use of any sleeping agent can easily become a difficult habit to break and may also interfere with the diagnosis of the real problem. I do not recommend using barbiturates because they are dangerous and habit forming.

146

Do not hesitate to make an appointment to review the situation with your primary-care physician, especially if you have a number of other symptoms or if you take several medications. However, if you want to try a few measures at home before seeking a medical evaluation, consider the following: For people who are having difficulty falling sleep, going to bed can actually be a stressful time of the day. Few things are more frustrating than "trying" to fall asleep and then tossing and turning for hours on end. In order to make your bed a place associated with feelings of rest and relaxation, leave it if you have not fallen asleep within twenty or thirty minutes, and then return when you feel more drowsy. Don't use the bed as a place to read, write letters, watch television, have arguments with your spouse, or finish the day's work. Going to bed and waking up at the same time—every day of the week— tends to reset the body's internal clock and normalize sleep.

Several of the easier-said-than-done recommendations of previous chapters are helpful in curing insomnia. Regular exercise blows the physiologic "all clear" whistle, as we noted earlier, and helps with overall relaxation. However, working out late in the evening can interfere with sleep, so morning or late afternoon is preferable. Laying off alcohol, cigarettes, and caffeine during the late afternoon and evening (or for good) may be necessary.

Dealing with any issues that are causing your sleepless nights may require an act of great courage. You may need to seek help from a good friend, counselor, or pastor to ventilate the problem and hear some constructive solutions. Indeed, the spiritual underpinnings of sleep may need the most attention. The ability to sleep peacefully may be a barometer indicating how well we have turned over our cares and concerns to God at the end of the day (and for that matter, through all of the waking hours). In chapter 12 we will consider how much we really believe God is in charge of the universe and our individual lives. For now, consider this observation of King David:

> *I will lie down and sleep in peace,*
> *for you alone, O LORD,*
> *make me dwell in safety.*

(Ps. 4:8)

ELEVEN

The Dark Night of the Soul

Drainer—The many faces of depression
Gainer—The many facets of treatment

One of the few detailed studies of chronically tired patients revealed that over half had psychological-profile scores that strongly suggested depression. (By comparison, *none* of a group of control patients without fatigue symptoms showed similar profiles.) This association does not indicate whether depression causes fatigue,
fatigue causes depression, or both are caused by a common underlying disorder.[1] In real life, all of these relationships are possible. In chronic fatigue syndrome (CFS), which we reviewed in chapter 6, for example, it is likely that fatigue and depression arise from the same infectious-immunologic disorder. On the other hand, when someone feels ill for a long time for any reason, some degree of depression is virtually inevitable.

DEPRESSION AND FATIGUE

This chapter will focus on depression as a cause of chronic fatigue—a relationship that is easily overlooked and undertreated. Most people think of depression primarily in emotional and psychological terms—feeling sad or even hopeless, having "the blues," or having a negative outlook about life in general. For the moment we will be looking at what the medical community calls "major depression"—an episode of disturbed mood lasting more than two weeks, not having an obvious medical cause, and manifesting a number of common symptoms. Traditionally, depression has been categorized as *situational (reactive)* or *biochemical (endogenous)*, although most depressed people seem to have some elements of each.

Situational Depression

Situational or reactive depression is a response to a major loss or reversal in life. The death of a loved one, the loss of a job, a business failure, a home destroyed by disaster, an unexpected diagnosis of a serious disease—all of these normally trigger a grieving response that has predictable stages. Indeed, ignoring or avoiding the grieving process can create new problems. For some, however, the reaction is severe and prolonged, interfering with normal activities and relationships for months or years.

A situational depression might be compared to a physical injury that doesn't heal. In minor injuries, we feel the initial pain, but within a predictable period of time, the injury heals, leaving only a small scar. In a severe injury, the pain will be intense, the repair process prolonged, and the scars more obvious or even disfiguring. Similarly, a major loss (especially the death of someone close) or rejection (divorce or separation, being fired from a job) will have a profound but foreseeable impact on emotions and behavior; suffering will be intense, the recovery process long and difficult, and the changes permanent. But in some cases, physical wounds do not heal; they remain open sores. This is caused not by the injury itself but by tissue disorders or by habitual picking at the wound. Similarly, a severe emotional wound may not progress toward healing because of pre-existent emotional problems or even biochemical tendencies toward depression. A few people become stuck at some point in the process, unable or unwilling to lay the issue to rest; they remain emotionally raw for months on end.

One elderly patient was beset by dozens of physical complaints, of which fatigue was the most profound. After working through her list of symptoms for several weeks, I began to talk with her about her emotional "weather," which was perpetually gloomy. She suddenly broke down in tears, sobbing over a son who had died more than fifty years earlier. Despite the passage of half a century, she had never returned to a point of equilibrium after her great loss.

In general, anyone who suffers a tragedy in life will benefit from the guidance and support of a counselor or group whose members understand the wound and the process of recovery. Good friends, of course, can be of great comfort, but those who know how the damage feels and how recovery progresses will be the most helpful. A number of years ago my wife lost two brothers in an airplane crash. While I and many others offered all of the comfort we could, a close friend whose brother died under similar circumstances understood the situation far better than any of us. Her help was the most valuable.

Biochemical Depression

Biochemical or endogenous depression has roots in the biochemistry of the brain. It also tends to have insidious beginnings, often generating a host of physical rather than emotional complaints. Of these, chronic fatigue leads the list, usually with a poorly defined date of onset. Disrupted sleep is very common as well, marked by difficulty falling asleep and staying asleep or in some cases by a desire to sleep all the time. Excessive appetite or loss of appetite and a collection of aches and pains (or numbness and tingling) in various parts of the body may also be a part of the package. Apathy, or a loss of interest in activities that were previously pleasurable, is very common. There may be less resistance to alcohol, drugs, or destructive sexual relationships. (These symptoms can be very much a part of a situational depression as well.)

Often biochemical depression seems to come out of nowhere. Someone who is progressing through life without any ongoing upsets may unexpectedly become weary, apathetic, or overtly sad. The process may last for a few weeks and then fade away, or it may drag on for months. Recurrences throughout life are common. Patients often refer to similar episodes beginning during the teen years (or even earlier), as well as similar stories in parents and siblings. This pattern strongly suggests a genetic and biochemical problem. In fact, current theory holds that a deficiency in one or more of the neurotransmitters—the chemical messengers necessary for communication between nerve cells in the brain—leads to the complex of symptoms seen in biochemical depression.

Episodes of biochemical depression can be effectively treated with nonaddictive medication, but ironically patients may offer considerable resistance when this idea is suggested. First of all, many people with these symptoms do not think of themselves as depressed. They're tired or they have insomnia or they have aches and pains everywhere, but they don't have an "emotional problem." I often tell people to think of themselves as having a "recurrent neurotransmitter deficiency," which sounds more like a treatable illness. Even so, they usually feel uncomfortable taking anything called an antidepressant. They worry that it will be addicting, like some sort of "upper." They don't want a crutch. "Normal" people solve their problems and get on with life.

In fact, antidepressants are not "uppers," and they have no addiction potential. No one sells them on the street, because they don't create any immediate euphoria. Ideally, there should be less stigma associated with taking antidepressants than with taking insulin for diabetes. In the right person, they gradually replace the depleted neurotransmitters, leading eventually to a sense of being back to normal without any artificial "buzz." After three to six months, they can be stopped, usually with no noticeable effect (although a certain number of people with chronic neurotransmitter problems need to continue medication indefinitely). Basically, if you don't need them, they don't do anything very noticeable.

The choice of an antidepressant should be made by

a physician who has taken a careful history and evaluated all of the options for treatment. Usually a single daily dose is taken at bedtime or in the morning, and gradual changes in the amount of medication are made over several weeks. The symptoms of depression do not miraculously disappear overnight, and three weeks may pass before any difference is noted. Usually the first problem to resolve is insomnia, a benefit that most fatigued people appreciate greatly. Even more gratifying is an improvement in energy levels, which often bring the depressed person to the doctor in the first place. As with any type of drug, side effects are possible. Some of the most common agents produce dry mouth (a sure sign that the drug has reached adequate blood levels). Sedation and changes in appetite may be experienced. (These are less common in the newer medications, such as Prozac and Wellbutrin.)

I mentioned earlier that most episodes of depression have some of the characteristics of both the reactive and endogenous types. Indeed, it is likely that every case falls somewhere on a spectrum between the purely biochemical and the completely situational extremes. For most depressed people, therefore, some combination of treatments is most effective. If the symptoms warrant, medication can help normalize mood, energy, and sleep. At the same time, a number of personal issues may need some work with an appropriate counselor. Unresolved pain from the past may need to be healed. Current relationships may be malfunctioning. The job or career may not be working out as planned, and vocational changes may be in order. Unhealthy attitudes and habits may perpetuate bleak moods. A relationship with God may need to be started or rekindled.

The Dark Night of the Soul

COPING WITH DEPRESSION

A number of other actions can help clear a depressive episode or at least contain any damage it causes. Keep in mind that choices made (or not made) during a depression may have long-standing repercussions that actually intensify the problem. If a depressed mother at home doesn't get out of bed, the general disorder that results will only make her outlook more bleak. If a negative mood results in some ill-timed remarks at work, a demotion or even the loss of a job won't improve the emotions one bit. One bad decision can lead to another, with an ever-worsening downward spiral of hopelessness and apathy.

Ongoing contact with family and friends is important because depressed people tend to withdraw from circulation. However, if the normal circle of cohorts consists of people with perpetually bad attitudes or substance abuse problems, staying home is a better idea. People in a depressed mood tend to be preoccupied with themselves (how bad they feel, how poorly they are doing compared with so-and-so, how rotten things have turned out, and so on). Sometimes looking outward and helping someone else solve a problem can be highly therapeutic. I routinely try to convince depressed people to look for an active, growing church if they don't belong to one already. Focusing on God (who never gets depressed), getting involved with some other people in a small-group study, and volunteering for a hands-on service project or two can work wonders or at least put people in a healing arena.

Working on some of the other drainers addressed in this book can help lift a depression, even if only tiny steps can be taken at any given time. Physical exercise, for example, has long been recognized as effective in improving mood. Changing dietary habits may be necessary. Getting rid of booze and cigarettes, which for many people are a false refuge from their unhappy emotions, may also be critically important. While suggestions like these are, once again, much easier to say than do, a skilled counselor or supportive group of friends can help move things along a little at a time.

Not all depression problems fall into the categories I have just described. There are other, more unusual and intense forms of depression that should be managed primarily by a psychiatrist. *Psychotic depression,* in which a person not only feels unwell but has delusions or hallucinations, must be treated immediately using specific medications. *Suicidal* people likewise need aggressive care by professionals well versed in intervention. *Bipolar* disorder (known more commonly as manic-depressive illness) consists of mood swings in two directions: manic episodes, in which a person feels outgoing, energetic, and literally "on top of the world" (but with terrible judgment); and depressive episodes, which are often horrendously bleak. The two phases may occur months or years apart, or they may swing unpredictably from one day to the next. Medical management of this disease is difficult but critical in order to prevent utter chaos in a person's life.

Maintaining balance while dealing with depression is obviously very important, since ultimately many types of care may be needed. Those who believe that every depressive episode is caused by neurotransmitter defects may place too much emphasis on drugs while ignoring important issues that are fueling the problem.

Others who feel that drugs simply mask the real problems (bad attitudes, habits, and relationships) may see very slow progress in physical symptoms, which are influenced by the neurotransmitters. Some Christians see depression strictly as a spiritual problem that should be addressed with Scripture, exhortation, and prayer. They tend to see drugs as a cover-up and intensely distrust anything resembling psychology. While this position is somewhat extreme, it is correct in one respect: Many professional therapists fail to address some of the spiritual aspects of depression.

SPIRITUAL DIMENSIONS OF DEPRESSION

Guilt, Repentance, and Forgiveness

Perhaps the most important issues are guilt, repentance, and forgiveness. Over the past quarter century, the need to acknowledge, confess, and repent for personal wrongdoing has become a highly unpopular subject in a culture steeped in concern over self-esteem and positive self-image. However, the Scriptures teach that we are from the first breath bent toward rebellion, toward being the god of our own universe.

We are born with a nature that cares desperately about how we look, how we're doing, how much we own, and whom we influence. It wants us to be in control. It wants to avoid blame or responsibility when something goes wrong. It tends to rationalize, excuse, and deny. When it runs the show, a lot of physical and emotional energy will ultimately be expended trying to satisfy it. A smooth veneer and some transient "highs" will be undergirded by a lot of effort. Burdens will be borne indefinitely, even when repressed.

However, within us is also another voice, one that is sensitive to absolute standards and the One who set them in place. It wants to do what is right, to feel clean and innocent. This voice is built into all of us, even those who have no formal training in spiritual precepts. The apostle Paul refers to people who had no direct contact with explicit moral laws but who "show that the requirements of the law are written on their hearts, their consciences also bearing witness" (Rom. 2:15). Our inclination to follow God's orders may be empowered by moral teaching beginning in the earliest years, or it may wither under the barrage of evil circumstances and the example of calloused people around us.

Ultimately, our spiritual welfare hinges on much higher stakes than simply believing that God exists or that our balance sheet contains more good deeds than bad. We must face the reality that our rebellion disqualifies us from having a relationship with God at all. No accumulation of good works or religious ceremonies on our part can bridge the chasm between each of us and God—a chasm that results from our wrongdoing and, to coin a word, our wrongbeing.

Each of us is thus faced with one of two options. First, we can continue to bear, both now and eternally, the consequences of our attitudes and actions that offend God. We miss the mark, both accidentally and deliberately. In his summation argument against humanity's claim to innocence, the apostle Paul argues forcefully that "all have sinned and fall short of the glory of God" (Rom. 3:23).

Second, we can choose to repent, to acknowledge

that we have nothing to offer God at all, and to accept all that he has to offer us: his payment of the overwhelming penalty each of us deserves. The first time this happens—when we understand that Jesus suffered and died so that we could be forgiven completely for all of our rebellion against God and when we surrender our lives to him—the experience is life changing, referred to in Scripture as a second birth (John 3:5–8).

When we take this critical step, we have literally chosen life over death, and much more: "Therefore, if anyone is in Christ, he is a new creation; the old has gone, the new has come!" (2 Cor. 5:17). God now actually dwells in us individually, in a way different from the presence of a general sense of right and wrong. This new birth and all that it entails is the ultimate energy gainer, because God is the ultimate source of all purpose and power for an infinite period of time.

So why do Christians, who have had this eternity-changing experience, still have problems like depression and chronic fatigue? Because the world and our physical bodies are fallen and because the "old nature" does not depart from the "new creature." In particular, the capacity and urge to do what is wrong or to ignore what is right can be contained, but it will not go away. The moment-by-moment relationship with God must be maintained and cultivated on an ongoing basis, much like breathing. Wrongdoing must be acknowledged for what it is, and forgiveness already provided by God must be experienced again, perhaps several times a day (or hour). Unfortunately, there are several common hindrances to all of the experiences of forgiveness.

Blaming, one of the most common human behaviors, has become a veritable pastime in American society. Without any training or prompting, children will bicker over "who started it" or "who broke it," pointing the finger in all directions when punishment may be at hand for a wrongdoing. This tendency does not necessarily disappear during the passage to adulthood. When tragedy strikes, when a project fails, or when some expectation (great or small) is not met, the question "Who's to blame?" follows immediately after "What's the damage?" Since we live in an age in which fixing blame can be highly profitable (especially when there is insurance money to be tapped), taking any or all responsibility for an unfavorable event can be a risky business indeed. We see today virtually no role modeling for mature acceptance of responsibility when something goes wrong.

Denying that we sin is a behavior closely related to blaming. If we find no one available to be the object of a pointed finger, we often cry, "It's not my fault." In some instances, dealing with issues in psychological terms lends credibility to this denial. If we perceive our wrongdoing to be a result of unmet needs or a poor self-image, we don't feel the need to repent.

Similarly, *denying that there is anyone to sin against* short-circuits the energizing process of dealing with personal wrongdoing. Our culture is permeated with a notion that the most important factor in a moral decision is whether it "feels right," with some secondary concern over whether anyone "gets hurt." Some churches proclaim that God is not nearly as concerned about our little imperfections as he is about the broad sweep of social injustice or the environmental destiny of the planet. Those in the New Age movement are convinced that we all are God (usually without realizing it) and that what we might call good and evil are but different sides of the same reality. In all of these quarters the idea of confessing and repenting before an ultimate authority in the universe has been relegated to the status of a medieval relic. But a euphoric view of self, on whatever basis, will remain in tension with everyday failures and aggravations.

False guilt is the flip side of denial. Accepting blame for events over which we have no control drains our energy and causes depression. The heavy but unrealistic weight of responsibility children feel when their parents divorce is a dramatic example. Equally severe is the guilt victims of abuse feel. Wives who are battered by their husbands, routinely accept responsibility for their wounds. (Indeed, the church has all too often given women the highly malignant message that allowing themselves to be clobbered every day fulfills a biblical duty of submission to their husbands.[2]) Children who are sexually abused and rape victims in general are all too often burdened with a powerful sense of guilt and shame, as if they somehow were to blame for the violence thrust on them.

In much less dramatic everyday circumstances, many people find a false sense of responsibility to be an energy drainer. Trying to live with other people's expectations of us (for example, to take on a new volunteer project when our schedule is already jammed) can lead to an erosion in energy.

The *inability to accept forgiveness* can be a major barrier even to those who are not dealing with denial or false guilt. Jesus may have paid it all on the cross, but some people believe that a righteous God would not want anything to do with them. My wife, Teri, has worked extensively with women who are dealing with negative emotions—especially anger and depression—in the wake of a past abortion. Many Christian women or those who have become Christians since having one or more abortions are unable to comprehend that God could forgive them for what they have done. Some carry for years the notion that if they are good enough for a certain period of time (usually five to seven years), they will be welcomed into a more intimate relationship with God.

Lack of Direction

Another spiritual issue related to depression is a *lack of a sense of direction.* Plodding through a daily routine, treading water, living week to week or month to month without sensing that anything significant is going on can contribute to any depressive episode. On the other hand, a meaningful and driving purpose that generates numerous personal goals is highly energizing. Consider, for example, the tone of the book of Ecclesiastes. King Solomon surveyed his magnificent surroundings and achievements with the bleak attitude that all of it was meaningless. Amidst all of his splendor, Solomon, like the tycoon Howard Hughes, had lost his bearings. Compare this with the excitement bursting throughout the book of Acts. The earliest Christians took their world by storm, rejoicing after beatings and singing in prison because their commission was so compelling.

The Dark Night of the Soul

Spiritual Warfare

A third spiritual issue related to depression is that of spiritual warfare, the unseen conflict between God and his enemies. Perspectives about this issue are often marked by extremes: people either dismiss it as fantasy or exaggerate it into distracting proportions. Jesus himself and the leaders of the early church acknowledged the influence of demonic forces in a variety of circumstances, and they stressed the importance of spiritual maturity in dealing with them. Those who have dabbled in occultism, trance channeling, hallucinogenic drugs, or overt satanism have set out the welcome mat for entities that are not interested in their well-being. Severe, relentless depression, among other manifestations, can result.

Even those who "fight the fight" as servants for God are not immune to the impact of the war on their minds and bodies. Elijah handed the prophets of Baal a humiliating defeat in a "praying contest" on Mount Carmel, a resounding public demonstration of God's authority (1 Kings 18). But within days he was running for his life from the enraged Queen Jezebel until he reached a point of total exhaustion and despair. "He came to a broom tree, sat down under it and prayed that he might die. 'I have had enough, Lord,' he said. 'Take my life.'" (1 Kings 19:4). Only after he received angelic nourishment and had some intense conversation with the Lord did his depressed condition improve.

Most people who have worked on the front lines of ministry have experienced unexpected episodes of oppression, where an invisible but palpable cloud seemed to settle over them. Confession of any wrongdoing, counsel, and prayer with others having maturity and insight is usually far more effective than any antidepressant medication in these situations.

Overall, a word to the wise is in order: *All* the avenues of treatment—medical, psychological, and spiritual—have their place, but the blend in each case will differ for each person or even change in the same person as time goes on. Don't be afraid to seek help in all areas. For further reading I highly recommend Minirth and Meier's book *Happiness Is a Choice*, which addresses all the components of depression in an informative and readable style.[3]

TWELVE

Stress and Distress

Drainer—Mental trench warfare
Gainer—The big picture

Throughout history physicians and patients alike have needed buzzwords to explain the symptoms and disorders that stump them. Although terms like "foul humours" and "miasma" are extinct and "It must be a virus" doesn't always fly, there remains a surefire, catchall cause of disease: *stress.* In recent years stress has taken the rap for nearly everything, including high blood pressure, low blood sugar, runny nose, headaches, heart attacks, cancer, canker sores, and especially fatigue.

How is stress related to fatigue? What is stress? How do our bodies physically respond to stress? How can we learn to cope more effectively with the stresses we face?

WHAT IS STRESS?

The identification and management of stress has become a booming industry in the past twenty years, as books, tapes, videos, and seminars have proliferated in an effort to help curb this apparent plague. Unfortunately, much of the discussion of this subject in the media, in doctors' offices, and over the back fence has been muddied by uncertainty over the meaning of the word. At least four concepts of stress abound in our culture:

1. Stress refers to dealing with unpleasant external circumstances. This is the most common understanding of the word. When people say, "I'm under a lot of stress right now," they most often mean that one or more areas of life have taken a downward turn or that they have so much to do in so little time.

2. Stress is an unpleasant internal response. When someone groans, "I'm really stressed out over this situation," they often mean that they perceive their circumstances as overwhelming or unbearable.

3. Stress is the body's response to a given challenge. When confronted with a situation demanding some action, our bodies activate several physiological responses known as the "stress response." If this response did not occur, meaningful activity (not to mention survival of the species) would be limited.

4. Stress is the ultimate consequence of our body's stress response. Much has been written about stress as a long-term disease that causes a wide array of symptoms and outright physical damage. Some authors have over-reached a bit by placing stress at the root of nearly every ailment, while others have more appropriately raised interesting questions about very complex interactions between mind and body.

All of these concepts have some degree of validity, but to avoid confusion, let's focus on the definition this book will use: Stress is *any situation that requires a person to act or change.* The event may be trivial (getting up to answer the phone) or profound (fighting off an attacker), pleasant (winning a contest) or unpleasant (being sued). The *stress response,* on the other hand, is a relatively stereotyped series of physiological events that enable a person to deal with the situation at hand.

HOW DO OUR BODIES RESPOND TO STRESS?

Typically the stress response includes a rise in blood pressure, an increase in heart rate and muscle tone, a dilation of the pupils, a shunt of blood to the brain and the skeletal muscles (which propel the body), and a concurrent diversion of blood away from the intestinal tract, which doesn't need as much at that moment in time.

Much of this physiological response is mediated by the powerful hormone adrenaline (secreted by the adrenal glands, which sit atop the kidneys), and by the sympathetic nervous system (a division of the autonomic nervous system, which regulates many bodily functions). Normally, after we meet whatever challenge we face, our bodies send out a physiologic all-clear signal, and our bodies return to baseline status.

We all have felt the rush of adrenaline after a near miss on the freeway or when hearing unfamiliar sounds outside the bedroom window. That "flight or fight" response is the body's way of coping with sudden and dangerous events. If our bodies did not automatically prepare for action, we could find ourselves unable to meet crises. Normally we respond much less intensely to something more routine, but without at least a mild physiologic change, we would collapse in a heap while getting out of a chair. Unfortunately, a number of things can go wrong with a complex system such as this.

Some people are physiological "hot reactors"—that is, they respond to every red light, phone call, or even a simple video game as if a saber-toothed tiger had just jumped through the window. Even when these people feel emotionally neutral, their blood pressure and pulse rate career up and down at the slightest disturbance. They may not realize that anything is wrong until their doctor tells them they have elevated blood pressures. Counseling or changes in lifestyle may change this pattern, but not always. How much of this is "hard-wired" genetically and how much is habit may be difficult to determine. Some people appear to be "addicted to adrenaline," feeling unsettled unless they are coping with one crisis or another.[1]

More often, problems arise because the "Murphy's Law" events of the day cause a physiologic eruption for hours on end. The alarm clock malfunctions, and you have to scramble to get to work on time. The kids are grouchy and dawdle through their cornflakes. Someone turned on the television or forgot to turn it off last night. The dog pooped on the carpet. One kid just spilled juice on the table, and the other can't find his shoe. Today's outfit was left in the dryer. No time for breakfast—grab the coffee and run. The traffic is piled up. All the parking spots are taken. The boss is waiting at the door, steam pouring from the nostrils, wondering why your report isn't ready for the new client. The phone won't stop ringing. And so it goes.

The body's preparations for "flight or fight" won't help here. You can't hit Mr. Dithers with a chair, saw the desk in half, or run down the street screaming at the top of your lungs. But your heart is beating more rapidly, your muscles tense up, your blood pressure soars, and acid pours into your duodenum. Your body does not send out an all-clear signal for the next eight hours. And what if arriving home is a literal jump out of the frying pan into the fire? If the place is a mess, the kids are fighting, and words best left unspoken get said, the physiological momentum will continue.

Some authors have argued that this relentless state of affairs contributes directly to the "diseases of civilization"—heart attacks, strokes, possibly even arthritis and cancer. For example, Meyer Friedman and Ray Rosenman in their book *Type-A Behavior and Your Heart* state that the "chronic excess discharge and circulation of the catecholamines (adrenalin and noradrenalin) . . . may be the chief factor in the total process of arterial decay and thrombosis."[2]

In a later article, Thomas H. Holmes and Richard H. Rahe developed a point system in an effort to gauge the amount of stress a person experiences over a given period of time. Heading their list was "death of spouse," which earned 100 stress points, with numerous other entries below it, such as starting a new job, moving, borrowing money, vacation, and Christmas. Their research suggests that if enough stress points are accumulated during a year, physical disease is more likely to occur.[3] The Holmes-Rahe Social Readjustment Rating Scale, as it is formally titled, has gained widespread acceptance as a measure of recent stressful events, although its capacity to predict disease is not cast in concrete.

Whatever effect a prolonged physiologic stress response has on the origin of disease, there is little reason to doubt that it contributes to fatigue. Having no all-clear signals in life is like running across a busy freeway with no safety zones. One particularly frazzled woman described her life as "one big left turn."

PERCEIVED THREATS

While stresses resulting from devastating crises or from life in an eternal fast lane can be exhausting, we must not ignore another vital ingredient in the stress equation: how we interpret what is going on. Many situations do put people under real stress: war, imprisonment, chronic abuse, or a lack of basic necessities such as food, shelter, or clothing will generate a long-term physiologic alarm in nearly anyone.[4]

But a lot of people who experience the same alarm every day, and who are chronically tired as a result, are not actually living under such terrible conditions. They may live in nice homes, eat plenty of food, and wear very decent clothes. They may even interact with civilized people every day. Unfortunately, however, they constantly *perceive* situations around them as threatening, and they react accordingly. What specifically is the threat? That *something will be lost or not gained.* What in particular? Some people fear losing safety, health, or basic comfort. Others fear losing income, position, loved ones, relationships, and self-esteem, resulting in a generalized alarm. Some people react intensely to situations that others might find mildly irritating or even interesting. When the response is extreme and specific, we refer to it as a phobia. Fears of heights or closed spaces are well-known phobias, but virtually anything—a dog, a bee, the dark—can set off a major alarm in the right person. Some unfortunate people live with intense fear, and all of the physical events that accompany it, in dozens of situations every day. Whether or not they verbalize it, they expect the worst. They feel that every car trip will end in a wreck. The neighborhood is full of malicious people. Every physical symptom is a sure sign of cancer, multiple sclerosis, or heart disease. Only two or three people in the world can be trusted, and the rest are either incompetent or malicious. The world is a very dangerous place, everywhere and at all times.

Yet in a very real sense, the world *is* a dangerous place. Turn on the evening news and watch the procession of terrorist violence, drive-by shootings, molestation, drug wars, pollution, and natural disasters. Nuclear warheads are poised only thirty minutes away, ready to be launched at a few moments' notice. AIDS is still spreading. Lots of bad things go on—but no one can live very well or very long with a relentless sense of imminent danger.

When fear is always at the wheel, our bodies will inevitably react. In response to a constant flood of adrenaline and a torrent of signals from the autonomic nervous system, we may feel chest pains, palpitations, shortness of breath, headaches, abdominal cramps—and most of all fatigue.

MANAGING STRESS

Since entire books have been written about stress management, we will discuss only a few important concepts. As with everything else related to plugging energy drainers, it is easier to know what to do than actually to do it. With that in mind, consider the following suggestions.

Making Changes

The core of all stress management is expressed in the famous prayer attributed to St. Francis of Assisi: "God grant me the serenity to accept the things I cannot change, the courage to change the things I can, and the wisdom to know the difference." If the pace of life is too intense, if there are too many demands from too many people, if too many bad things seem to be happening all at once, the first challenge is to decide what needs to change *externally* and *internally*.

External changes. Although altering your circumstances may seem impossible, never assume that things cannot change. Take a careful look at what you *can* do.

Is the neighborhood getting too crowded or noisy or dangerous? Is the drive to work too long and irritating? Then what can be done to change these conditions? If all else fails, what will it take to move?

Is your boss hard to work with? Is the work unsatisfying, boring, demanding, or pointless? Are your co-workers deadbeats or overly aggressive? Then what can be done to change these conditions? If all else fails, what would it take to work somewhere else?

Do you face constant financial pressure, with too much month at the end of the money and creditors calling day and night? Then what can be done to increase income or decrease expenses? What payment problems need to be renegotiated? If all else fails, should you consider filing for protection?

Stress and Distress

Do you face endless noise, arguing, and bad attitudes at home? Are your kids out of control? Is your relationship with your spouse dead in the water, lukewarm, or hostile? Then what can be done to change these conditions?

Internal changes. Unfortunately, many decisions intended to change your circumstances are made without considering *all* the options and most importantly without checking *what needs to be changed inside.*

Elizabeth had a lot of problems when she came to the office. She was thoroughly exhausted and was having a lot of headaches and stomach cramps. Some of her co-workers smoked, which really bothered her nasal allergy. Her boss demanded a lot and seemed to be on her case more than necessary. Along with a medical evaluation, she agreed to enter counseling just as she was beginning her third job in eighteen months.

During her counseling sessions, Elizabeth talked about her problems with employers and co-workers. As she described her conversations with them, it became apparent that she had strong ideas about how things should be run and that she felt quite free to express them. In addition, much of what she saw as an independent work style more often boiled down to overt noncompliance: she didn't want to do what the boss wanted done. The consequences of her expectations and actions were the main ingredients of the stress in her life, and her frequent job changes didn't improve matters at all.

Energy Drainers, Energy Gainers

Elizabeth's solution to her work problems was to quit and go somewhere else. The same game plan has been duplicated by all too many spouses dissatisfied with the home front. When the going gets tough, the tough get going—out the door in search of someone else. A string of distraught partners, damaged kids, and busy attorneys follows, as the endless search for "relief from stress" (caused by the person's own bad decisions) continues. Some with serious financial problems have tried out the same inappropriate "solutions." When pressures reach the boiling point, they walk away and leave others holding the (empty) bag.

What about stress related to the demands or needs of others—the projects at home, the committees at church, the social events on the calendar? In a subsequent chapter we will review the dynamics of overcommitment, but for now please note that changing an overwhelming "activity debt" also requires some internal decisions. What (or whom, other than spouse and kids) do you need to give up in order to see some improvement in the quality of life? What lies behind the inability to say no to the next person who wants something done? Need for approval? Pride? Some of each? Out of all of the things to be done, which are the most important? How many can be done by you and you only?

We also need to look at how we make changes. A sudden and drastic change in lifestyle may make for an interesting sitcom episode, but in real life the consequences may create more havoc than the original problem. We may need to honor some of our earlier commitments. We may need to phase out of some of our activities gradually. Careful and persistent working

174

through relationships and job assignments at work will be more productive than sudden demands for total change. In the financial realm, planning changes a step at a time—especially while communicating your intentions to creditors—will yield more fruit in the long run than finding a consolidation loan, borrowing more from the relatives, or simply bailing out by declaring bankruptcy.

The bottom line is this: It takes courage to make necessary external changes and wisdom to deal with necessary internal changes.

Reviewing Our Perspectives

This brings us to the *most* important aspect of stress management: changing our internal perspectives, expectations, and response patterns. If we are constantly feeling stressed and distressed, our *interpretation* of the sights and sounds of life may need to be retooled.

One of the problems inherent in the Holmes-Rahe stress-rating scale is that it doesn't deal directly with the mindset of the person experiencing the event. "Death of spouse," for example, is given the highest number of stress points on the scale. In most cases, indeed, this will be a highly distressing, unsettling event that profoundly affects the remaining years of the survivor's life. But what if, for some reason, the survivor is actually relieved when the spouse dies?

_____

David had suffered a serious mental deterioration over a three-year period. At first he couldn't remember where he left the keys or his glasses. Then he began making errors in the checkbook. When he began a household project, he rarely finished it, leaving it for others to clean up. He became increasingly irritable with Mary, his wife of fifty-two years, accusing her of stealing things when he couldn't find them.

Over several months, the situation relentlessly worsened. David became confused and agitated, especially at night. He almost started a fire when he put a plastic dish on the burner and then forgot about it. He would get up at four o'clock in the morning to rattle through the house, emptying drawers and files. He became convinced that family members had been plotting against him for several years, and he didn't hesitate to tell them what he thought about it.

David's doctor prescribed some medication to help him relax and sleep better at night, but he only became more unsteady on his feet, and the drug had to be discontinued. David became incontinent. Not only did his pants need changing and washing throughout the day, but his accidents began to appear all over the house as well. Mary finally came to the office one day to seek some help. She looked and sounded weary, frustrated, and overwhelmed by the unmanageable toddler that her husband had become.

Some time later David slipped and fell, breaking a hip. The surgery necessary to repair it went well, but while still in the hospital, a large clot dislodged from his leg and passed to his lungs. This major pulmonary embolus, as it is called, proved to be catastrophic, and he died shortly thereafter. David's death actually lifted some major burdens from Mary, and she found it less stressful than losing her relationship to him over the previous months.

What are the attitudes and orientations that ultimately matter the most in stress management? Since a perceived threat generates much of the stress response, I would like to propose a basic framework of three definitions that affect our perception as well as three practical ways to reduce the internal alarms.

Who is in charge? We need to define clearly and contemplate daily who is in charge of our lives. Does God rule over us and our circumstances? If we believe that God doesn't exist and that the universe is governed only by complex laws of cause and effect, then we have good reason to feel stressed. Does God care about our lives and is he involved in the day-to-day details of our existence? Some people believe that God is too busy with the grand scheme of the universe and the flow of history to attend to the details of our lives. After all, does the commander-in-chief of the armed forces know that the newest recruit just sprained his ankle? This notion of God's disinterest has been debunked in J. B. Phillips' classic book, *Your God Is Too Small:*

> Whatever a man's reaction may be to the idea of the terrific "size" of God, the point to note is that his comment is this: "I cannot imagine such a tremendous God being interested in me," and so on. He "cannot imagine": which simply means that his mind is incapable of retaining the ideas of terrifying vastness and of minute attention to microscopic

177

detail at the same time. But it in no way proves that God is incapable of fulfilling both ideas (and a great many more).[5]

We rarely admit that we believe God can't handle the vast sweep and the details at the same time. But even though we may not say it, we often act as if we are in charge, as if God couldn't possibly handle our circumstances. And sometimes we don't *want* God dealing with our everyday affairs. After all, who knows what demands he might impose on us if we really acknowledged that he is in charge of us at all times?

Assuming, however, that we believe that God can and does get involved in the details of our lives and that his intentions are good, we must take another step. Through repeated contemplation and prayer we must allow the truth that God is in charge to be driven deeply from the intellect through the emotions and into the physiologic reflexes, where it shapes the way we respond to situations. Such a lifelong process must be what the apostle Paul described as the renewing of the mind: "Do not conform any longer to the pattern of this world, but be transformed by the renewing of your mind. Then you will be able to test and approve what God's will is—his good, pleasing and perfect will" (Rom. 12:2).

Who are we? The second thing we need to define is who we are. On what do we base our self-concept? A preoccupation with the nurturing of our self-esteem has been so heavily promoted by the "me generation" that some authors have blasted any discussion of self-awareness as unbiblical. Yet like it or not, we all walk around with *some* set of assumptions about who we are, and these assumptions hold a direct line to the autonomic nervous system.

Is our self-concept grounded on a stable understanding of our relationship to God or is it built on the fragile whims of our culture? All too often, our identity is blown in every direction by feedback from other people and by cultural expectations.

If we yield to society's pressure to achieve success and power, we can soon drive up our heart rate, boost our blood pressure, turn on the stomach acid, and drain our body's energy. On the other hand, if we have established a relationship to God and understand that we are loved and significant, then we can use our energy to accomplish more useful purposes in God's kingdom.

Who or what will upset us? We need to decide who and what will be given permission to "ring our chimes," to push our emotional buttons. The list should be short, consisting primarily of those to whom we are most deeply committed. Our children will nearly always be on the list during the years they are young and dependent. In some cases, they stay on the list far too long.

For many years my grandmother was a worrier; she would fret about everyone's safety and health, including her own. Fortunately, her quick wit and sense of perspective held the reins on this tendency until she was well advanced in years. When she was ninety-two, however, she suffered a serious illness that left her memory severely impaired, and that removed nearly all restraint from her highly developed skill of worrying. As a result, she lives with an uncontrollable and urgent concern for the safety of her children, two of whom are grandparents themselves. Within a few minutes after one of them leaves her home, she feels agitated and will call them repeatedly until she knows they have made it home. The intensity of this worry has taken its toll on her and others as well.

The deep feelings between spouses and between parents and children will inevitably generate strong emotions throughout life. Beyond these important relationships, however, who else can push your emotional button? Your employer? The driver who cuts you off on the freeway (with gestures at no extra charge)? The slow tellers at the bank? Government officials? Your noisy neighbor?

I have a patient with a volatile blood pressure that is very difficult to reduce. Because his body language on several occasions suggested that something was bothering him, I probed to see if some personal issues might be playing a role. He denied any major conflicts at work or home, but he finally confessed that he becomes very agitated whenever he reads about a new Japanese acquisition in the United States. This anger is rooted in his combat experiences during World War II, and rather than putting his animosities to rest, he has allowed himself to become "cranked up" emotionally and physiologically on a regular basis. I kidded him a little about being the American equivalent of the legendary marooned Japanese officers discovered on desert islands three decades after Hiroshima, still ready for battle. When I asked him if his agitation was worth all the miseries and medications, he replied, "Not really, but I can't stop it." Unfortunately, he has cultivated this attitude for so long that nothing short of a miracle will free him from it.

Not only do we need to decide *who* will ring our chimes but also *what* will do it. When you face a situation that makes you tense, when your muscles tighten and your heart starts pounding, ask yourself whether the situation is worth the energy and emotion being squandered. Is this situation one that is important enough to get upset over? Is it a life-threatening matter? Does it affect the outcome of the human race? Will you remember what the fuss was about next year or even next week?

I write best when I'm under pressure. But when the deadline approaches, I tend to flare up when the computer malfunctions, when I can't find a reference, or when the phone rings once too often. I need to keep in mind that when the deadline is met, I'll forget the stress, but my children will not forget the fuming they overheard—and the more irritated I sound, the more intensely they will remember.

For times like this, we have a mandatory "time out" rule in our home: anyone who is overtly bugged by an inanimate object must get up and do something else for ten or fifteen minutes or until the storm blows over. Disturbances between people are another story—they are talked over on the spot if possible. We try to abide by a ground rule that no "thing"—whether it be a car breaking down, a temperamental appliance, a surprise fix-it project in the house, an assignment that's overdue (including this book), or an animal that "does a number" on the carpet—is worth straining, draining, and possibly shortening the lives God has given us. A lot of times we actually succeed.[6]

Releasing Stress

In addition to reviewing our perspectives, we can also practice three types of stress release.

Psychological releases. We need to program some time-outs and safety zones into our lives. Sometimes we gravitate toward these automatically. I taught myself to play guitar during hundreds of fifteen-minute study breaks over a ten-year period. I didn't do this as a matter of self-discipline; I just enjoyed how I sounded, as bad as it was at first. Sports, hobbies, and other diversions all can serve the purpose of blowing the physiologic all-clear whistle, especially if the activity involves laughter. Fifteen minutes spent with a book of Garfield cartoons or a half hour of "The Cosby Show" can recharge the batteries for the remaining responsibilities of the day.

On the other hand, any diversion can get out of control, interfering with more meaningful and productive activity. Witness the great American couch potato, with glazed eyes riveted to the boob tube for hours on end. Note the compulsive gambler or shopper or bar-hopper, whose search for recreation has become fruitless, if not destructive. Here the time-out from the pressures and responsibilities of life becomes a time-out from living at all. Looking for the ideal balance between tackling problems with a vengeance and getting away from them for a while is a lifelong search.

Physical releases. We need to become involved in activities that quiet down the adrenaline flow and the sympathetic nervous system. We already mentioned *aerobic exercise* (chapter 7), which has the added benefit of improving the general health of the body. A strenuous workout, especially at the end of a long work day, is an excellent way to blow off steam and forget about the day's hassles. More passive activities include a soak in a *hot bath or spa,* which helps relax many of the muscles that have tightened up during the day. Even more relaxing is a good massage, if an appropriate masseuse is available. (Married couples should note that massages often lead to other stress-reducing activities.) Finally, a good night's sleep can put the most intense situations into perspective.

What about medications to relax? The most widely used "attitude-adjustment" drug is, of course, alcohol. While an alcohol habit can lead to chronic fatigue (chapter 9), an occasional glass of wine with dinner or an occasional beer with friends can enhance an already pleasurable moment. But the risks and benefits need to be weighed in every situation. Do you use alcohol as a quick fix for a bad mood when more fundamental problems need to be dealt with? Will people (particularly children or teenagers) draw inappropriate conclusions about the role of alcohol in their lives from watching their parents or relatives use it on a regular basis? Does your ability to converse meaningfully end after a drink? Are you going to drive shortly after "happy hour"? Most importantly, has downing a drink or two become a daily ritual, a regular habit that you feel you need? The last question is the most important. When you feel emotionally drawn to drink, when alcohol is no longer a take-it-or-leave-it option, you need to consider avoiding it altogether.

What about prescription drugs to relax? The benzo-diazepines (Xanax, Valium, Ativan, Tranxene, and Librium, among others) are highly effective at producing immediate calm. But there's a catch, as many know all too well. They can easily become a habit deeply rooted in both mind and body. Those who have taken one of these drugs for weeks or months at a time become accustomed to the emotional time-out they create. They will also undergo intense physical symptoms (including convulsions in some cases) if they stop taking the medication abruptly. Withdrawal is a major project, requiring a very slow reduction of doses over several days or weeks, possibly in a hospital setting. Dealing with the physical symptoms of going "cold turkey" from narcotics is an easier job than helping someone cut their ties from benzodiazepines. In general, these drugs should be reserved for short-term use in a crisis situation.

A newer agent, buspirone (Buspar), has been used to treat chronic anxiety suffered by many people who feel long-term stress. Its effects are much milder, and so far there are no reports of addiction. Whether this medication is appropriate for a given situation is a matter to consider with your physician or a psychiatrist. Ideally, medication should be used for a defined and limited period of time, during which the more intense issues of life can be sorted out with a counselor or pastor. It is, indeed, difficult to solve problems when you always feel as if you're about to jump out of your skin.[7]

What about meditation? For the past two decades, various techniques based upon Hindu or Taoist mysticism, especially Transcendental Meditation (TM), have been pitched to materialistic Westerners as tools to manage stress. While the specifics vary, nearly all of these involve "clearing the mind" of its assorted hassles by repeating a word (or mantra) over and over, or by staring at a complex pattern (called a mandala), or by breathing and moving in very specific patterns. The persistent meditator is said to benefit from a more controlled stress response, lower blood pressure, greater creativity, more energy, and so on. (More ambitious programs claim to enable their disciples to walk on hot coals, regulate all sorts of otherwise unconscious bodily functions, and even float through the air.)

Several years ago, after TM promoters began telling their story to the world, Harvard physiologist Herbert Benson argued in *The Relaxation Response* that any benefits derived from meditating had nothing to do with magical mantras and mystical patterns; they simply resulted from sitting quietly for several minutes, breathing slowly and repeating a word—any word would do—several times.[8]

I agree with Dr. Benson—up to a point. The discipline of sitting quietly for twenty or thirty minutes a day undoubtedly has its benefits, but the "mind flush" produced by endless repetition of a word or phrase is a poor substitute for the biblical concept of meditation: contemplating with the conscious mind the attitudes and deeds of the God who created it. Let me suggest a more sound approach.

Spiritual releases. Too often a "quiet time" consists of a blitz through a few chapters of Scripture, often churning to keep pace with this year's "Through the Bible in a Year" program, followed by the pressured reciting of a laundry list of prayer requests. (You can tell I speak from personal experience.) There is nothing wrong with these activities, but they won't necessarily calm your spirit.

Consider sitting for several minutes in a comfortable room, or even somewhere outdoors with a nice view, with the phone off the hook and the television off. Take a few deep, slow breaths, and let a few of those tense muscles loose. Find a favorite verse or two and think about it—and nothing else. What does the verse say about God? What is God trying to say to you? What is there here to be thankful for? And so on. Let God take your mind where he wants. Later on, after this time, you can study the verse or the passage surrounding it in a commentary or whatever. For now, let the communication flow between you and your creator.

This is only one way that spiritual refreshment can impact on stress and distress. A time of worship with others drives the ideas that renew the mind deeply into the emotions and affects all sorts of reactions later on. Prayer reorients our limited perspective to God's eternal, infinite perspective. Ministering in a practical way to someone else who needs help takes our attention off our gripes and problems. A small group (Bible study or otherwise) that accepts, supports, exhorts, and laughs a lot in a well-defined safety zone of acceptance can serve as a weekly oasis.

These are all good and worthwhile things to do, but they are easier to agree with than to implement. You probably will need to do some active pruning to make room for these oasis times. Will there be false starts and misfires? Yes. But what else is new in our fallen world? Like everything else that fights fatigue, the benefits of these spiritual releases from stress and distress will usually be evolutionary rather than revolutionary.

THIRTEEN

Slow Leaks

Drainer—Daily aggravations
Gainer—Course corrections

We noted earlier that chronic mental and emotional fatigue is frequently a major component of the total fatigue picture. Usually this type of fatigue is caused by everyday irritations that may not seem to be major issues. However, when several are at work at the same time, we can become significantly fatigued. Consider these ten common slow leaks that drain our energy.

Overcommitment—Too Many Irons in the Fire

(I'm writing this segment primarily as a memo to myself. If anyone else cares to listen, be my guest.) Many times over the past decade Teri and I have tried to set a date for a night out by ourselves or with close friends, but when we looked at our schedules and responsibilities, we found no available time for three weeks. We have on other occasions scheduled two or even three activities in far-flung areas of Southern California on the same date. Invariably when such a day actually arrives and the little squiggles on the calendar have caused us to drive all over creation, we have looked at each other and groaned, "*Who* made up this schedule?" The answer is always the same: *We did!*

Like many of our friends, we wear several hats in a number of different arenas. We have daily and fundamental responsibilities to each other, our children, and our home. Years ago, after seeing James Dobson's original Focus on the Family film series, we committed ourselves to make time with our children a serious priority, and we have generally done so, whatever else has happened. In addition, Teri works with crisis pregnancy centers all over Southern California and travels extensively to speak about post-abortion syndrome. I have a busy primary-care practice, which alone could consume most of my waking hours, as well as a number of ongoing medical staff assignments at a local hospital. I serve on the board of directors of a major pro-life organization in Southern California. I have helped provide ongoing CPR training in connection with a Rotary Club to which I belong. We both prepare music and lead worship at two churches on a regular basis. We both have ongoing writing projects. We both need to read continually to stay current in our respective fields. We both try to follow our own advice about exercise. We both need, but too infrequently make, uninterrupted time to read the Scriptures, meditate, and pray. And the children have their own activities that require time and transportation. We occasionally like to sleep at night.[1]

All of these are very good and satisfying projects. But very often we feel out of control because the "activity debts" arising from promises we've made are colliding with one another. Life then becomes a series of brush fires, with the hottest and the closest flames getting the most attention. More than once I have complained about doing a half-baked job on a number of projects, rather than an excellent job on a few.

We mentioned previously some reasons why several plates may be in the air at once. We don't want to disappoint people. We may feel flattered when someone wants or needs us for a project we care about. A little pride may lurk in the background. We may fall for the dangerous delusional thought, "No one can take care of this problem but me," especially if it's an emergency. We may make a promise and write a fateful notation in the calendar without an honest evaluation of the time and effort required to fulfill the obligation.

Treatment. Dealing with the cluttered calendar is usually a lifelong battle. When someone asks you to do something, say the all-important phrase, "I'll get back to you shortly" and then ask yourself some serious questions. What really will be involved in this commitment? Why is this important? Are the basics (relationship to God and family) going to suffer as a result? If you are married, think carefully about filling another one of those boxes on the calendar without checking with your spouse. Coordinate your calendars weekly, if not daily. ("You scheduled us for what? I've got us down for something else!")

Most importantly, have the courage to say no when it's appropriate. Realize that you can't possibly do all the wonderful things you would like to do—even if you had ten lifetimes. Understanding your limits and drawing boundaries are acts of humility, not laziness.

Undercommitment—Too Few Meaningful Activities

In contrast to the overcommitted, some people attend only to the most basic needs of life. They are stifled, and usually tired, because they lack the energizing purposes and goals that would take them beyond the four walls of home. I see this especially in the people who find themselves adrift after retirement, having little on which to focus other than their growing list of ailments. These people represent a huge underutilized resource in our society.

Treatment. Pray, asking God to show you what you can do besides attending to everyday routines. Consider projects in your church, a local hospital or nursing home, the neighborhood, or even in some distant country. Which of your skills could assist someone else? Can you teach a disadvantaged person something you know (even if it's simply how to read)? You may change his or her life. Is there a nursing home in town? Many people who are confined there would be overjoyed to have a visitor on a regular basis. Is there a crisis pregnancy center in your community?[2] These ministries providing "shoe-leather" assistance to women in desperate straits are always in need of volunteers for lots of projects. Is there a prison or jail nearby? Prison Fellowship can put you to work in all sorts of significant activities that make a significant difference in inmates' lives.[3]

Your mission is not to change the world. But if you help change the world for one or two people, you'll definitely feel better as well.

Slow Leaks

Clutter—Accumulated Stuff of Life

Somewhere buried deep in the human psyche, right next to the primal urge to acquire things, is an equally powerful reluctance to let go of them. Unfortunately, our gradual accumulation of possessions is like an indoor overgrowth of weeds, which will suffocate us unless it is periodically pruned. A home or apartment crammed from one end to the other with "treasures" and trash is a major energy drainer. (Anyone who loves to wander through new model homes on a Sunday afternoon usually feels jealous of the fabulous decorating. In fact, most of the attractiveness is derived from the lack of clutter, which is easy to maintain because no one lives there.) Likewise, a cluttered desktop at work sends out the message that we are out of control. (This is another memo to myself.)

Treatment. Just as you can't do everything, you can't *keep* everything either. (Notice the pattern emerging throughout this book?) Undoing the clutter can be an energizing experience. And after you've done it, you may not even miss the dearly departed junk. Do one room or closet at a time so that you don't feel overwhelmed. (Save the garage for last.) Turn on some upbeat, unsentimental music—this job requires ruthlessness at times.

When looking through your closet, weed out all clothing that hasn't been worn for a year or more. Goodwill Industries will find it a nice home. Have you looked at those magazines from last year? You won't this year either. How about those cans of paint with just a little bit left? Chuck 'em. Do you need to keep *every*

191

piece of artwork Johnny brings home from preschool? Not unless you want to be buried alive by the time he reaches junior high. Of course you want souvenirs of his activities, so pick the best of the lot, preserve them carefully and faithfully, and toss the rest.

What about the drawer full of video tapes of shows recorded for viewing at some later date? I still have all eighteen or whatever hours of "War and Remembrance" scattered over several tapes, and I have yet to watch the first ten minutes. That growing library of programs may be nothing more than another form of clutter. You can probably rent most of them at the video store for two bucks any day of the week.

A more difficult question: What about all those books? We *hate* throwing away books, because someone might need something in one of them sometime, right? But a two-volume history of Turkey? That math textbook from college? The *Reader's Digest Condensed Books* from 1967? The repair manual from the car you sold five years ago? We love books—but not all of them have to be within reach forever.

Another tough area is the kids' rooms. Most children have a phenomenal tolerance for clutter. To a reasonable degree, if what they strew about is confined to their own quarters, a little slack will conserve a lot of everyone's energy. (Remember: Few children have ever died of dirty-room disease.) However, a little gentle persuasion may be needed to train them in at least a few habits of civilization. More drastic measures such as short-term confiscation may be necessary if their possessions are left all over the house. Taking Barbie or G.I. Joe hostage for a few days can help reinforce the importance of cleaning up one's own things, but you'll probably need to write a ransom note to remind them that something is missing.

Once some order is restored, notice how good it feels. To maintain that positive emotion, remember that the "circular file" is one of your best friends.

Debt—The Paper Chain

Getting into debt is as easy as gaining weight, and getting out is as hard as losing it. I'm convinced that the urge to shop is one of the primal drives of humanity, right alongside self-preservation, food, and sex. We have to buy things on a regular basis to survive, but buying also happens to make us feel good. And our present society is absolutely crammed with nifty items that not only thoroughly satisfy the basic needs (food, clothing, and shelter), but also offer all sorts of experiences, prestige, and stimulation. Unless you live in a cave, hundreds of these wonderful enticements beckon every day.

In the good old days, most people stopped buying things when there was no more money. Unfortunately, we presently have many ways to bypass that little inconvenience. Most of them are small plastic cards that for some idiotic reason make us act as if we had money in the bank. Why not enjoy that item now, rather than waiting until we have the money to pay for it?

And so it comes to pass that after but a few years of adult life, it is easy to owe much to many. Those whom we owe also like to be paid, and they care little about the effort we have expended juggling bills, answering hostile phone calls, racing to the bank with the paycheck to cover all those hot checks, arguing with our spouse (if we have one) over how little money there is and why, and worst of all refinancing. They just want to be paid. So large amounts of energy and time drain away in exchange for something that very often isn't generating much pleasure any more.

Treatment. Getting out of debt requires about the same approach as losing weight. We need to face some basic realities. First, we need to understand that God owns everything. Therefore, we don't "own" our worldly resources; we only manage them. Second, there is always more to be bought than we could ever buy, so we must stop somewhere. Third, we need to understand the flow of our own income and expense needs. Some of us hate to deal with the gory details of what we actually spend and what our financial status actually looks like. Denial is as powerful a force in spending as in eating.

We need to pick out a resource, whether a counselor or a book, develop a plan, and then stay with it. The problem will not go away overnight, and no one wants to live like a Tibetan monk for very long. More than one financial planner has suggested taking the smallest debt first and paying it off while maintaining the minimum requirements on the others. Each account sent to zero can be the occasion for a "retirement party." Also, if you make yourself accountable to someone else, that person can help you stay on course when you are tempted to give up or go on a spending spree. Again, fear of losing face can be harnessed to help accomplish what willpower cannot.

These few paragraphs are only an introduction to the many resources you can find about managing your money. Larry Burkett, founder of Christian Financial

Resources in Atlanta, for instance, has written excellent resources about money management and debt busting.[4] I also recommend Ron Blue's book *The Debt Squeeze*.[5]

Workaholism—Breaking the Fourth Commandment

Workaholism is a special form of overcommitment—in one direction. I have asked some tired people about their work schedule and have found myself equally tired listening to the answer. One middle manager in a high-tech corporation told me how his boss had insisted on a seven-day work week (in which the boss himself was not participating) until a colossal project was completed. This highly educated engineer, who could analyze anything, hadn't a clue about why he was so tired and was stunned by my rather blunt response: a written prescription for one day off per week.

Hard-driving corporate types are not the worst violators of the Fourth Commandment. The self-employed, especially those with small businesses, are always vulnerable in this area. They frequently don't feel secure enough to forget about their enterprises for a day, carrying them home in their brains after business hours and dragging reluctant family members into their private sweatshops as well. Second on the list for workaholic risk are care givers: physicians, psychologists, social workers, and pastors. Since the dimensions of human need in any community are virtually limitless, all who meet needs for a living can easily burn out with exhaustion if they are always "on call."

195

Treatment. Obviously diligence, responsibility, and excellence are noble goals for corporations and small businesses; family enterprises can be a very meaningful activity for all concerned; and reaching out to those in need is a high calling. *But, remember the recurring theme:* There is always infinitely more work to be done than we could ever do; there are more needs to be met than we could ever meet. Therefore, we must draw decisive lines across which work will not be given a toehold. The line may be a place (such as home, unless the office is at home) or more importantly a *time*. It is extremely important to have a minimum of one day per week (Sunday very often) in which you do not work. When Jesus noted that the Sabbath was made for man and not man for the Sabbath, he was talking about more than religious observances.[6] God *commanded* a day off every week for the sake of the survival and sanity of the humans he loves.

In our family it is very easy for work to creep in at all hours of the day and night. Teri works half of the week out of the home, but calls come in during most times of the other half as well. When she is off hours, the answering machine is her most valuable asset.

When I'm on call for our medical group, I have no choice but to be a well-paid slave. But after I hand the baton to the next person in the rotation, I really don't want to hear about anyone's symptoms or medications until the next appointed time.[7] If an acquaintance who has my home number calls with a medical problem, Teri nicely but firmly refers him or her to my on-call colleague. Otherwise, once I hear about the problem (in other words, "Tag, you're it!"), I feel obliged to take care of it. If someone pulls me aside in church with a question about this or that pain, I ask them to make an appointment; otherwise, I can't think about worship and they get a distracted, incomplete answer. (One of my partners has another approach: When someone asks him about symptoms at a party or the store or church, he replies, "Well, take off your clothes right here so I can examine you!" So far he hasn't had any takers.)

The day off, by the way, is not the time to clean the garage or check off the first five items on the "Honeydo" list. It should be a time to refresh, reflect, recreate, worship (especially if it's Sunday), spend time with people we care about. Sometimes it's necessary to escape to a park, beach, zoo, movie, museum, or whatever puts a distance between us and the brush fires. For those who struggle with the idea of a day to recharge the batteries, I highly recommend Tim Hansel's book, *When I Relax, I Feel Guilty*.[8] While the title might suggest Sunday supplement fluff, Hansel has some very provocative thoughts about work and recreation. Don't miss the part about five-minute vacations.

The TGIF Syndrome—Why Work?

Whenever a local newspaper prints a story about an instant millionaire in the state lottery, I'm fascinated by an inevitable consequence: The first thing the big winner does is quit his or her job. I spent a few college summers working at a mortgage banking company, and I was struck by the cloud of gloom that hung throughout the office on Monday morning and gradually lifted as the weekend approached.

Obviously it's necessary for most of us to be gainfully employed. However, if work generates no greater satisfaction than a paycheck every other week, then five or six out of seven days will be spent fighting fatigue. Thinking about the lottery winners should generate an important question for all of us. If we had a substantial income from some other source, would we continue the job we are doing now?

Treatment. We need to reflect once in a while about what our work accomplishes in the scheme of things. Who benefits from what we do? If the answer is "no one in particular," and if after a most careful assessment we decide that our work is, in the words of King Solomon, "all vanity," then we need to do some creative thinking about other ways to spend forty or more hours a week.

On the other hand, before blowing off steam about your "lousy job" and making noises about quitting to do who knows what, a little precautionary prayer and wise counsel are in order. Jumping from job to job may be symptomatic of a deeper lack of contentment or of a permanently critical and ungrateful attitude. Furthermore, perhaps the workplace is an arena into which God has called you to be salt and light. I'm certain that the apostle Paul did not see tentmaking as his primary mission in life—but he didn't belittle it either, since it ultimately gave him a certain level of independence as he pursued his goals of preaching and teaching.

Raising Small Children—Always on Call

Some of the most tired people who visit me at my office are the parents of infants and toddlers. Back in my early days of practice, I used to ask this routine but naive question to women with kids draped all over them: "Do you work?"

Finally one of them shot back, "No, I just sit around eating bonbons all day!" I suddenly realized how insulting this question was. Anyone who has assumed responsibility for small children for more than five minutes, and taken the job seriously, understands that this is one of the most challenging tasks on earth. (Since the mother is most often the one who assumes this assignment when the children are small, I will refer to her in this segment. But what I have to say also applies to the stay-at-home father.)

I always warn first-time parents to be ready for a few revelations when they take their wiggly bundle home for the first night. Although our son Chad was born by Caesarean section (an event that puts an additional drain on the mother), we felt well prepared for our first solo flight with him at home. We were well educated and motivated. Chad was a very wanted child. And we had very supportive grandparents helping us. To top it off, in my residency clinic work, I was busy telling young parents "how it's done."

But all through his first night in our bedroom, Chad made lots of noises and rustled around in his bassinet. Each sound snapped our eyelids open as we wondered whether or not he would wake up fully for a feeding. The next night we moved him into an adjoining room, realizing that he would let us know when he was hungry. That worked well, but he still let us know when he didn't appreciate the room service in the dead of night, the diaper changes, the rocking, and the lullabies. He didn't notice how sore Teri was, how sleepy we both were, and how hard we were trying. He cried anyway, with that newborn cry that sounds so irritated and dissatisfied. (The power of that sound to move adults to action is, of course, programmed into the human species as a means of survival for infants.)

It was during a few of those memorable nights that we began to feel "put upon," a signal to let him cry for fifteen minutes while we calmed down and got things into perspective before trying again to get him to sleep. We both realized how bad things could get for people in less favorable circumstances—for single moms, for young couples with limited resources, or for anyone whose feelings about the whole child-rearing process were mixed. How easy it would be for the combination of unpleasant feelings, chronic fatigue arising from sleepless nights, and unending responsibility to escalate into child abuse or neglect.

As Chad grew into toddlerhood and his sister Carrie entered the picture, I was working to build a medical practice and to contain its demands, while Teri struggled with some different issues. What do you do when the kids have left the room and you're still watching "Sesame Street"? How many times can you hear "The Happy Dump Truck" record before you start singing it—when no one else is around? What does it mean when the high point of your day is watching reruns of "The Bob Newhart Show" while the kids lie down for a nap? Why bother to clean up the house when it automatically returns to total disorder within thirty minutes? Is it possible to be attentive to the needs of small children without your brain turning to Cocoa Krispies?

Lack of sleep, lack of adult conversation, and lack of any sense of forward motion (except watching the kids get bigger) drains vast amounts of energy from the most talented, motivated, and dedicated moms. In addition (and probably most importantly), lack of recognition for the job being done drives many into unnecessary despair as they picture their childless friends advancing in seemingly glamorous careers and wonder what kind of idiots they are for staying home. (Alas, the media and the feminist movement have for the past generation reinforced the notion that staying home to raise children is a less desirable option than working outside the home.)

Treatment. There are *lots* of things that can help plug this very important energy drain. First, for the person who stays home:

1. Develop some appropriate expectations for this season, this surprisingly brief passage (that seems like an eternity at the time). Life is not "passing you by." There will be many, many years ahead to carve your niche in society, if that is what you are called to do.

2. Remind yourself of the importance of this job, even if no one else seems to appreciate it. These years are very significant for both you and the children, and they can be fascinating years as you observe the changes and growth happening every day during otherwise routine events.

3. Who says the mind has to go numb for several years? What books do you want to read besides *Goodnight Moon* and *The Runaway Bunny*? What was your major in high school or college? No one said you couldn't keep learning or continue taking courses at a local college when the children get a little older.

4. Cultivate relationships with other adults (of the

same sex). Regularly scheduled times of grown-up conversation are critical, and your spouse may not be able to meet all of your needs in this area. This is especially critical for the single parent, who is bearing all of the responsibility single-handedly.

5. Find the best baby-sitters in the area, and reward them well (if you can) so that you may have some time-outs on a regular basis—not for errands, but for brief periods of personal refreshment. Going out with friends or getting your nails done or just taking a walk alone is both legitimate and necessary. When cash is short, a resourceful alternative is the baby-sitting co-op, where child care is swapped on a barter system among several people. If you are blessed with loving grandparents nearby, let them spoil the kids for a few hours (or even overnight) while you get a break.

If you are a single parent, you have some of the greatest challenges of all, since there may not be another adult in the vicinity to share the child-rearing load with you. All of the principles mentioned in this chapter apply even more to you, and you will have to take strong measures to maintain your sanity and balance. Don't be afraid to make your needs known at your church. Most importantly, don't be too proud to accept what is offered.

If you are the husband of the stay-at-home care giver, you have a critical role in maintaining her sanity. She needs to hear that she is important and desirable. She needs adult conversation, not more prattle from the television. She needs someone to take charge of the kids for a while, even while she's right there in the room. She needs to be dated and even taken away for a weekend if you can arrange it. She needs to be brought flowers and sent cards for no particular reason. She needs to be encouraged to develop her mind and her skills; caring for the kids one night a week while she goes to a class would be a courageous act on your part and would also give you an intense appreciation of the magnitude of her daily work. (In the less common arrangement of working mom and stay-at-home dad, the same principles apply—perhaps minus the flowers.)

Above all, those who raise children need to stay on their knees, because no one has all the answers, wisdom, and energy needed for the job—but God does. Don't forget: The process will teach you more than any other experience about your relationship to God, who is the ultimate loving parent.

Conflict on the Home Front

During the first few years of our marriage, we enrolled in a "couples' communication" class sponsored by our church. While we felt that the material in the course seemed almost painfully elementary at first, we also learned how easy it is for the most trivial discussion to inflict damage, unintentional or otherwise. Subsequently I have watched dozens of couples or entire families talk to each other in my office—where everyone is more likely to be a little more cautious—with relentless tones of disagreement and disrespect.

More recently this type of ongoing verbal trench war has been broadcast weekly in the popular television sitcom, *Roseanne*. (The intent is for the characters' banter to be funny, of course, but the role modeling is terrible.) The ongoing prodding and accusing, putdowns and sarcasm, arguing and in some cases physical fighting creates an atmosphere that is draining and polluted. Since the patterns are usually ingrained and automatic, the combatants may be aware only of their constant dissatisfaction and fatigue.

Treatment. This is one of the toughest energy drainers to plug because ideally two or more people need to recognize the problem and the need to learn communication without verbal clubs. (However, one highly motivated person can model some constructive patterns for the others.) An astute counselor can facilitate this process, but so can any couple or family whom you have observed to have their act together in this area. If your church offers couples' communication classes, be the first in line to sign up. For a sneak preview of some patterns to cultivate, consider the following ideas when dealing with any issue in the immediate future.[9]

1. Avoid questions that begin with "Why ..." ("Why did you do this?" "Why did you say that?") "Why" questions are a verbal attack and will always provoke a defensive answer, unless the other person decides to hunker down with the famous response, "I dunno," or the sarcastic one, "I guess I'm just an idiot."

2. When lodging a complaint, use "I" statements that say how you feel, instead of "you" statements that tend to sound like accusations. Example: "You don't listen to me," which calls for a rebuttal, doesn't work as well as "I feel really uneasy when your eyes are on the TV when I'm talking."

3. Avoid the words *always* and *never* when discussing an issue. "You always say that!" implies that the other person has a character disorder, whereas "I remember this same argument, and I don't agree with it

because . . ." makes a more specific point. In addition, avoid rehashing old business during a current topic, unless historical verification is absolutely necessary. A comment like, "This is just like five years ago . . ." treads on thin ice, because another issue has just been opened. Draw comparisons from the past very carefully and specifically if they are needed to make a point.

4. Timing is important when bringing up issues. No one can carry on an intelligent discussion when the television is blaring, the dog is barking, the kids are crying, and the phone is ringing. The very end of the day may bring out the worst in everyone because fatigue and irritation are amplified. Sometimes, if the topic is important enough, a visit to a local restaurant for a meal or a cup of coffee will provide a more relaxed and civilized arena for the discussion.

These techniques may prevent a lot of aggravation, but they assume that the people involved respect each other and want improvement. In some relationships and families this is not the case, and the daily warfare is rooted in true animosity, often with very deep roots of mistrust, anger, and even outright abuse. When this much damage has been done, a lot of time, effort, and accountability (to a counselor or peers) will be needed to bring about healing. The process will be rewarded with much energy regained, among other things.

Garbage In, Garbage Out—
The Mind As Trash Barrel

In a day when consumers read product labels and work to keep themselves free from additives and pollutants, we often demonstrate an impressive lack of selectivity about what enters our eyes and ears. We have all heard the nauseating statistics about children seeing umpteen thousand murders on television by the time they're seventeen years old. Lurking below that statistic is a much deeper and broader exposure to brain toxicity from *many* sources.

Even the best newspapers earn their keep by reporting what went wrong yesterday. The worst, which guard the supermarket checkout racks, seep with the dregs of human behavior (not to mention their "amazing stories" of aliens, monsters, and voices from beyond). Television and films, which compete very successfully with real human contact in the contest for our time, have become more extreme in their subject matter, offering a scarcity of wisdom or positive role modeling. Popular music has become the subject of controversy recently, and for good reason. Flipping through the album covers in the rock-and-roll (and especially the heavy metal) bins of any music store is like taking a trip through Dante's inferno—and that's before the music is played. A very solid contingent of the CD and tape market consists of material preoccupied with death, violence, and unusual uses for genitalia.

Pornography and slasher films continue to do big business, especially with their availability through neighborhood video stores. They have also invaded nearly every hotel room in the nation through pay-for-view cable services. Aside from their grossly immature understanding of sex and their predatory attitude toward women, "adult" films contain the vilest material available for human consumption. The *Friday the 13th* and *Nightmare on Elm Street* films, and others like them, are just like pornography, except that episodes of extreme violence rather than random sex interrupt the idiotic dialogue. It is a pathetic commentary on popular culture that the murderers in these series (hockey-masked Jason Vorhees and razor-gloved Freddy Krueger) have actually become popular icons. Needless to say, hours spent watching people copulating indiscriminately or hacking each other to pieces are guaranteed energy drainers. Sadly, the video habits of careless adults have exposed millions of children to these sights and sounds—and they will never forget them.

Treatment. To set some guidelines, use discretion and discipline. Every individual and family has different standards for handling the media. Some do very well by unplugging the television, canceling the newspapers, and doing radical things with leisure time such as reading, talking, pursuing a hobby, playing games, or making music. At the other extreme are those who are indiscriminate or even habituated to violent or sexually oriented material.

No one wants to live in Fantasyland, and serious looks at real problems are a necessary part of responsible citizenship. But the content and tone of materials to which we subject our minds (and our children's) needs careful review. Is there any value in what is about to be read, heard, or seen? Is there anything to be learned, discussed, or prayed about? If younger people are going to see a well-made but intense video at home, is there a responsible adult around who will fast-forward through any particularly unpleasant spots and then discuss the movie when it's all over?

For most people, knowing what they're getting into

at the outset is half the battle. Unfortunately, movie and television reviews and even the movie-ratings system often fail to predict how the material and tone will affect us. Some newspapers print capsule movie reviews from the PTA, tipping off parents about the appropriateness of a film for younger viewers. The Catholic church has its own rating system that predates the current MPAA ratings (Motion Picture Association of America), and the *Movieguide*, published by Ted Baehr, is an excellent resource for information about both content and *orientation* of films and some plays. (*Movieguide* also offers some hot tips on excellent but poorly publicized films, such as the delightful *Babette's Feast*.)[10]

What about time spent in the car? Does the radio play an endless litany of bad news or foul jokes from "shock radio" disc jockeys? Most cities and towns are within range of at least one Christian radio station, and most of these now offer programs that are both thought provoking and uplifting. High-quality broadcasts such as "Focus on the Family" and "Insight for Living," among many others, have displaced much of the rambling commentaries so common twenty years ago. Better yet, a cassette player in the car is a valuable asset because so many excellent tapes are available from churches, bookstores, or the radio itself. (I routinely record "Focus on the Family" for listening in the car.)

What about music? Above all, the content and orientation of the words are of critical importance. What are the lyrics saying? How does the overall sound affect you? Some people claim they listen to the death-and-violence groups "just for the beat" while ignoring the words (which, arguably, are often unintelligible). But the message generally gets through one way or another.

People whose taste runs to the more energetic sounds might appreciate alternatives like Petra or First Call or artists like Amy Grant and Michael W. Smith. A useful source for information about contemporary music is Menconi Ministries, which publishes an excellent quarterly magazine *Media Update,* plus books, tapes, and videos that are both informative and balanced.[11]

The bottom line is this: Like anything else in life, the drainers (in this case, the garbage in) seem to happen automatically. The gainers (which encourage, educate, and edify) need to be worked for. The apostle Paul's advice deserves our consideration on a daily basis: "Whatever is true, whatever is noble, whatever is right, whatever is pure, whatever is lovely, whatever is admirable—if anything is excellent or praiseworthy— think about such things" (Phil. 4:8).

Unmet Expectations and Desires

"Things aren't turning out the way I had hoped," the story goes. The degree, the home, the job, the raise, the spouse, the new toy just aren't producing lasting contentment. The restless search for the next item that might bring satisfaction continues—and the fatigue accumulates.

So what else is new? Centuries ago King Solomon surveyed all that he had acquired: unimaginable wealth, political superiority, worthwhile building projects, education, and the sexual satisfaction of 1000 partners. Yet he was still not a happy camper:

I denied myself nothing my eyes desired;
I refused my heart no pleasure.

My heart took delight in all my work,
and this was the reward for all my labor.
Yet when I surveyed all that my hands had done
and what I had toiled to achieve,
everything was meaningless, a chasing after the
wind;
nothing was gained under the sun.

(Eccl. 2:10–11)

Treatment. At some point in life, a major issue must be settled: Is contentment (not complacency) created internally or is it the result of "how things are going"? What dictates mood: circumstances or a forward-looking, others-oriented, stable attitude sustained by God working on the inside? Solomon himself answered the question:

> A man can do nothing better than to eat and drink and find satisfaction in his work. This too, I see, is from the hand of God, for without him, who can eat or find enjoyment? To the man who pleases him, God gives wisdom, knowledge and happiness, but to the sinner he gives the task of gathering and storing up wealth to hand it over to the one who pleases God. (Eccl. 2:24–26)

Unfortunately, like most of the other treatments for chronic fatigue we have mentioned, knowing the principles is not the same as living them. I have seen too many tired, dissatisfied people who have known the Bible well. For this treatment to work, another one of those *daily* disciplines needs to happen—*daily*. The process involves thinking about who God is, and what he has done, and what he thinks is important—*daily*. The entire book of Psalms begins with this idea:

> *Blessed is the man*
> > *who does not walk in the counsel of the*
> > > *wicked*
> *or stand in the way of sinners*
> > *or sit in the seat of mockers.*
> *But his delight is in the law of the LORD,*
> > *and on his law he meditates day and night.*
> *He is like a tree planted by streams of water,*
> > *which yields its fruit in season*
> > *and whose leaf does not wither.*
> *Whatever he does prospers.*
>
> > > > > *(Ps. 1:1–3)*

The image of the tree is powerful, one worth comparing to our own daily experience. It is solid, stable, productive at the right time, drawing life constantly from the waters nearby. And we can be like it when we are turned in the right direction and when we keep our Designer's instructions constantly before us.

Notes

Chapter 1
The (Usually) Unanswered Question

[1] A perverse tradition in medical training refers to an unusual disorder as a "great case," even when it spells disaster for the patient.

[2] The stories in this book are told to illustrate typical scenarios related to chronic fatigue. Some of them are composites of two or more people, and the names have always been changed.

[3] According to the *National Ambulatory Medical Care Survey: 1975 Summary,* published by the U.S. Department of Health and Human Services (PHS 78-1784), fatigue was the seventh most common symptom in primary-care offices at that time. It is doubtful that this complaint will ever fall from the top-ten list.

    More recently, a survey of 1,159 consecutive patients at a broad-based acute-care clinic and internal-medicine office showed that 24 percent of the patients considered fatigue to be a major problem, whether or not they expressed it at the time of the visit. (Kurt Kroenke et al., "Chronic Fatigue in Primary Care: Prevalence, Patient Characteristics, and Outcome," *Journal of the American Medical Association* 260 [1988]: 929–34.)

[4] Kroenke's study noted no particular variations in prevalence of fatigue based on age, educational background, or race. However, women reported the symptom at a higher rate (28 percent) than men (19 percent).

Notes

Chapter 2
Energy and Fatigue: Some Basic Principles

[1]Paul C. Reisser, Teri K. Reisser, and John Weldon, *New Age Medicine* (Downers Grove: InterVarsity Press, 1988).
[2]When no medical disease has been revealed by a medical history and physical exam, additional studies (such as laboratory tests) will reveal an unexpected physical disorder about 10 percent of the time.

Chapter 5
Misunderstandings About Causes of Fatigue

[1]It is worth noting that the human body closely monitors changes in blood glucose in order to secrete an adequate amount of insulin. A large intake of simple sugar can raise blood sugar rapidly, leading the pancreas to believe that a huge amount of food has just entered the body. If it actually overshoots the mark (an event not easy to prove without frequent blood testing), blood sugar may drop too quickly, leading to a variety of unpleasant but *transient* symptoms.
[2]William Crook, *The Yeast Connection: A Medical Break-through* (Jackson, Tenn.: Professional Books, 1984).
[3]Ibid., 28.
[4]Corinne Allen, "Allergies, the Disease of the 20th Century," *Nutritional News*, Dr. Allen's publication.
[5]Ibid.

Chapter 6
The Special Problem of Chronic Fatigue Syndrome

[1]Walter C. Hellinger et al., "Chronic Fatigue Syndrome and the Diagnostic Utility of Antibody to Epstein-Barr Virus Early Antigen," *Journal of the American Medical*

Association 250 (1988): 971–73. This article focuses particularly on the antibody to the so-called "early" antigen (that is, a portion of the virus that stimulates an early immune response). A number of different types of antibodies against EBV can be measured, but this particular type was thought to be the most specific indicator of the chronic EBV syndrome.

[2]Gary P. Holmes et al., "Chronic Fatigue Syndrome: A Working Case Definition," *Annals of Internal Medicine* 108 (1988): 387–89.

[3]Ibid., 389. I have paraphrased some of the CDC's medical terminology.

[4]Information in this paragraph was derived from summaries of presentations given by Dr. Arthur Komaroff of Harvard Medical School and by Dr. Margaret Tipple of the Division of Viral Diseases at the Centers for Disease Control at the first national CFS conference held in San Francisco on April 15, 1989. Reported in the newsletter of the National Chronic Fatigue Syndrome Association: *Heart of America News* (Spring 1989): 1.

[5]Jesse Stoff and Charles Pellegrino, *Chronic Fatigue Syndrome: The Hidden Epidemic* (New York: Random House, 1988).

[6]The three groups are

1. National Chronic Fatigue Syndrome Association
   919 Scott Avenue
   Kansas City, KS 66105 (913-321-2278)

2. Chronic Fatigue Immune Dysfunction Syndrome Society
   P.O. Box 230108
   Portland, OR 97223 (503-684-5261)

3. Chronic Fatigue and Immune Dysfunction Syndrome Association
   P.O. Box 220398
   Charlotte, NC 28222-0398 (704-362-2343)

Notes

[7]Karyn Feiden, *Hope and Help for Chronic Fatigue Syndrome: The Official Book of the CFS/CFIDS Network* (Englewood Cliffs, N.J.: Prentice Hall, 1989).

Chapter 7
Getting Off It and Getting On with It

[1]Kenneth H. Cooper, *Running Without Fear* (New York: M. Evans and Company, Inc., 1985), 104–5. This effect is described in much detail in Dr. Cooper's books about aerobics, including *The Aerobics Program for Total Well-Being* (New York: Bantam Books, 1983) and *The New Aerobics for Women* (New York: Bantam Books, 1988).

[2]Despite the usual heavy breathing involved, sex really doesn't qualify as aerobic exercise. Horseback riding does not qualify either, unless you happen to be the horse.

[3]By the way, being handicapped, chronically ill, or elderly is *not* an automatic disqualification for regular exercise.

[4]This is discussed in considerable detail in Kenneth Cooper's book *Running Without Fear*.

[5]Many hospitals now offer cardiovascular screening programs that include a treadmill along with an overall assessment of the risk of coronary artery disease.

[6]Arguments against routine screening treadmills on all people at a certain age are based on calculations suggesting that the number of procedures (and their cost) required to discover one unsuspected heart problem are unacceptable. These considerations regarding cost-effectiveness are useful in designing strategies for large populations but less helpful when caring for an individual patient who is seeking specific advice.

[7]Many of these are available, with a wide range of intensity. A few seem preoccupied with close-ups of female anatomy, such that much of the heavy breathing by male viewers isn't the result of moving muscles.

Notes

Chapter 8
Nutri-Symptoms

[1]Please note that most physicians have not been trained to be experts in dietary details. Furthermore, there are appropriate qualifications for giving dietary advice, and the initials R.D. following one's name (denoting Registered Dietitian) usually indicate that reasonable information is forthcoming. Unfortunately, all sorts of self-styled "nutritionists" are more than willing to dispense bizarre advice and expensive supplements. Don't be afraid to check credentials.

[2]For more detailed information, see the current edition of *Jane Brody's Nutrition Book* (New York: Bantam, 1987). Ms. Brody, health columnist for the *New York Times*, covers a lot of ground, keeps her information interesting, and has done her homework. This is an excellent resource.

[3]Eighty percent of all diabetes cases are the adult-onset form, which does not require insulin and usually responds primarily to weight reduction. Furthermore, obesity is a known risk factor for cancer of the uterus.

[4]Jane Brody, *Jane Brody's Nutrition Book* (New York: Bantam, 1987) and Jane Brody, *Jane Brody's Good Food Book* (New York: Bantam, 1986).

[5]Sonja L. Connor and William E. Connor, *The New American Diet* (New York: Fireside Books, 1986).

[6]Covert Bailey, *Fit or Fat* (Boston: Houghton Mifflin, 1978).

[7]The medical problems associated with extreme weight gain or loss will overshadow the issue of fatigue, which is usually present as well. Those who are beset with these conditions need specific treatment by well-trained clinicians.

217

Notes

Chapter 9
Side Effects

[1]Drugs, like any other product, have both generic names and brand names. Usually the brand name is better known, even though the generic form, if available, may be less expensive. (Unfortunately, generics are not always of the same quality and effectiveness as brand name medications.) In order not to be seen as giving an endorsement, this chapter will identify a medication by the generic name, with one or more brand names following in parentheses. For example, someone with the aches and pains of the flu might consider taking acetaminophen (Tylenol) for relief.

[2]For those who are reading this material after the year 1990, please note that new medications (or entire groups) will now be available. Some of the comments in this chapter may be dated, but I have never claimed to foretell the future.

Chapter 10
Mr. Sandman, Bring Me Some Sleep

[1]J. Christian Gillin and William F. Byerly, "The Diagnosis and Management of Insomnia," *The New England Journal of Medicine* 322 (1990): 239–48.

Chapter 11
The Dark Night of the Soul

[1]Kurt Kroenke et al., "Chronic Fatigue in Primary Care: Prevalence, Patient Characteristics, and Outcome," *Journal of the American Medical Association* 260 (1988): 929–34.

[2]An excellent but disturbing treatment of this subject may be

found in the book *Battered into Submission* by James and Phyllis Alsdurf (Downers Grove, Ill.: InterVarsity Press, 1989).

[3]Frank B. Minirth and Paul D. Meier, *Happiness Is a Choice* (Grand Rapids: Baker, 1978).

Chapter 12
Stress and Distress

[1]A more detailed picture of this type of person is offered in Archibald D. Hart, *Adrenalin and Stress* (Waco, Tex.: Word, 1986).

[2]Meyer Friedman and Ray Rosenman, *Type-A Behavior and Your Heart* (New York: Knopf, 1974), 178.

[3]T. H. Holmes and R. H. Rahe, "The Social Readjustment Rating Scale," *Journal of Psychosomatic Research* 11 (1967): 213–19. J. Petrich and T. H. Holmes, "Life Change and Onset of Illness," *Medical Clinics of North America* 61 (1977): 825–38.

[4]It should be noted, however, that human beings have an amazing ability to adapt to adverse situations—up to a point. Much depends on the inner orientation to life and to circumstances.

[5]J. B. Phillips, *Your God Is Too Small* (New York: Macmillan, 1961), 41.

[6]Probably the greatest challenges to our rule were provided by our dearly departed 1981 Volkswagen Vanagon. Known lovingly as "The Money Pit," "Der Fuehrer's Revenge," and "*!@ + *!!"—this vehicle drained us of time, resources, and energy for five years.

[7]I would not be honest if I did not mention that some people seem physiologically unable to function without some sort of sedative on board. For whatever reason (genetics, upbringing, habit, or all of the above), their central nervous system is like an engine that idles too fast, and

Notes

no amount of counseling or insight seems to help. These people will find whatever is necessary to slow it down, and a controlled prescription is definitely safer than alcohol or some illegal concoction.

[8]Herbert Benson, *The Relaxation Response* (New York: Avon Books, 1975).

Chapter 13
Slow Leaks

[1]Lest anyone think from this list of activities that we are hopeless workaholics, I might add that we also have enough of a hedonistic streak left to take the phones off the hook and enjoy a video movie, a game, or an outing with the kids whenever possible.

[2]If you want to locate a local crisis pregnancy center, call or write the Christian Action Council, 701 W. Broad Street, Suite 405, Falls Church, VA 22046 (or phone 703-237-2100). Other organizations operate such centers as well.

[3]For information about local projects, write or call Prison Fellowship Ministries, P.O. Box 17500, Washington, D.C. 20041-0500 (or phone 202-265-4544).

[4]Christian Financial Resources, 601 Broad Street, S.E., Gainesville, GA 30501 (404-534-1000).

[5]Ron Blue, *The Debt Squeeze* (Pomona, Calif.: Focus on the Family, 1989).

[6]Mark 2:23–28.

[7]I'm continually grateful that I work in a medical group in which I can let someone else worry about the patients at predictable times. Likewise, I always wonder how solo practitioners, especially those serving rural communities, maintain their sanity when they can rarely escape being on call.

[8]Tim Hansel, *When I Relax, I Feel Guilty* (Elgin, Ill.: David C. Cook, 1979).

Notes

[9]Strictly speaking, an issue is any subject about which one or more people are concerned and about which they want to talk. An issue can range in significance from the way the toothpaste is squeezed (center or end?) to the deepest crisis between people.

[10]To subscribe to *Movieguide* (currently $30 per year and worth it), write to Good News Communications, P.O. Box 9952, Atlanta, GA 30319.

[11]Al Menconi Ministries, P.O. Box 969, Cardiff by the Sea, CA 92007-0810.